THE SPANISH FLU EPIDEMIC AND ITS INFLUENCE ON HISTORY

For Bob, Mark, Muriel, Paul, and in memory of Karen.

THE SPANISH FLU EPIDEMIC AND ITS INFLUENCE ON HISTORY

Stories from the 1918–1920 global flu pandemic

Jaime Breitnauer

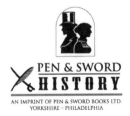

PEN & SWORD
HISTORY

AN IMPRINT OF PEN & SWORD BOOKS LTD.
YORKSHIRE – PHILADELPHIA

First published in Great Britain in 2019 by
PEN AND SWORD HISTORY
an imprint of
Pen and Sword Books Ltd
Yorkshire – Philadelphia

ISBN 978 1 52674 517 0

Typeset in Times New Roman 11/13.5 by
Aura Technology and Software Services, India
Printed and bound in the UK by TJ International

Pen & Sword Books Ltd incorporates the imprints of Pen & Sword
Archaeology, Atlas, Aviation, Battleground, Discovery,
Family History, History, Maritime, Military, Naval, Politics, Railways,
Select, Social History, Transport, True Crime, Claymore Press,
Frontline Books, Leo Cooper, Praetorian Press, Remember When,
Seaforth Publishing and Wharncliffe.

For a complete list of Pen & Sword titles please contact
PEN & SWORD BOOKS LIMITED
47 Church Street, Barnsley, South Yorkshire, S70 2AS, England
E-mail: enquiries@pen-and-sword.co.uk
Website: www.pen-and-sword.co.uk

Or
PEN AND SWORD BOOKS
1950 Lawrence Rd, Havertown, PA 19083, USA
E-mail: Uspen-and-sword@casematepublishers.com
Website: www.penandswordbooks.com

Contents

Author's preface

There is some sweet irony attached to the fact that, in the year I decided to write a book about the worst pandemic in human history, my own son spent time in the grip of serious illness. While his malaise was not viral, it did involve many trips to the GPs, hospitals and various specialist clinics that we often take for granted as part of a robust public health system.

While researching and compiling the various personal accounts in this work, I was simultaneously navigating our family's own path through both medical and social support systems. Although that was complex and not always satisfying, learning about the varied experiences of the millions of people worldwide who suffered during the pandemic that became known as Spanish flu made me eternally grateful for the simplicity that is access to comprehensive and affordable medical care.

In Britain, the NHS was part of the legacy of Spanish flu, alongside two world wars. After the ravages of the first forty-five years of the twentieth century, the government made a decision that a strong country would offer its citizens free-at-point-of-use healthcare and a welfare net to catch those at risk of falling off the bottom rung. The positive impact – and sense of relief it brings those who need to use it – cannot be underestimated.

There has been a flurry of interest in Spanish flu and its legacy over the last few years as the centenary of the Great War was marked. Many volumes of work have been produced, either academic in nature or fictionalized accounts of historical fact. It was my hope with this work to marry the two, offering a creative re-telling of the experiences of real people, giving an authentic face to the many tragedies that unfolded.

Just as public healthcare in the UK was in part a legacy of this pandemic, each country touched by flu between 1918 and 1920 (and it was pretty much all of them) was shaped in some way by their suffering. As well as walking you through the history of the time I have aimed to leave you with some understanding of the impact on each locality, and the wider global community.

J S Breitnauer, December 2018

Prologue

The month before war

Standing in the sunshine on Appel Quay, a broad avenue running alongside the river Miljacka in central Sarajevo, Bosnia, 19-year-old Gavrilo Princip reached into his jacket to check for his gun. It was 28 June 1914 and the avenue was crowded, full of people here to see Archduke Franz Ferdinand, heir presumptive to the throne of the Austro-Hungarian Empire and inspector general of its army. Having annexed the Slavic state of Bosnia in 1908, Ferdinand was here to inspect the troops charged with keeping order.

The crumbling Ottoman Empire had stepped away from 400 years of rule in Bosnia in 1878, when a series of uprisings forced it to cede administration of the region to Austria-Hungary. This change of governance was not well-received by increasingly independence-minded political groups and a heavy hand was used to bring swift order and control. It would be 30 years before the annexation was formally agreed in 1908 and those three decades were characterised by struggle for recognition by the varied people of the land – Catholic, Orthodox and Muslim. It was within the context of this rising tide of nationalism and an increasingly longing gaze for the territory from neighbouring Serbia, that Princip was born.

Standing amidst the relative opulence of the capital's main street, Princip thought of his home village of Obljaj in Western Bosnia, sandwiched against the Croatian border and the forests of Herzegovina. Known colloquially as *vukojebina* or, 'the place where the wolves fuck',[1] the people of this windswept, desolate landscape were occupied with survival. It was here Princip was raised in acrid poverty. He thought of his father, Petar, a Serbian farmer and postman who struggled to keep his family fed. He remembered his eight brothers and sisters, six of whom died as babies, and his mother Marija's resigned but loving face as she cared for him through yet another illness. Sickly but inquisitive, Princip lost himself in books and set out for Sarajevo aged 13 to get a better education. He remembered that journey now, traversing hills, fording watercourses and crossing farmland, his feet feeling the ghostly aches of a hike that would have taken the best part of a week.

Along the way, he met all sorts of people with varied heritage but sharing a common trait – they were unhappy with their lot in life. They were unhappy with living to survive, with the oppression that comes from being governed by a separate nation state and Princip felt this acutely.

Princip fingered the cold metal of the 9mm Browning pistol in his pocket and felt the heat radiating from the stone of the three-storey building behind him. Even though it was still early, the sun was bright and the day was going to be warm. To his right, in the distance, he could see the motorcade moving slowly along the crowded street and he considered what would happen next.

One of six conspirators planning to murder the visiting Archduke, Princip had been placed in position five along the motorcade route, a fail-safe in case things did not go to plan. Ahead of him were Bosnian-Muslim Muhumed Mehmedbašić, and Bosnian-Serbs Vaso Čubrilović, Cvietko Popović, and Nedeljko Čabrinović. Further up the river by the Kaiser Bridge, Trifko Grabež waited as a sixth man and leader Danilo Ili, a member of Serbian Nationalist group the Black Hand, looked on. Each had a weapon – a bomb or a gun – and each was ready to take a life for a better Bosnia.

Princip wondered how history would remember them after this day. Next to his gun was a vial of cyanide – he had no plans to find out for himself. Turning sharply away from the sun he caught sight of his reflection in a shop window. A slender teenager with a toothbrush moustache and ill-fitting suit, he didn't stand out in the crowd. He wondered if, after his death, people might flock to his grave the way they did with Bogdan Žerajić, a 22-year-old Serb medical student from Herzegovina who had martyred himself in 1910 for the nationalist cause. Princip himself had spent many nights holding vigil there, thinking about how he could influence what he saw as an ideal goal, a united Yugoslav province. Because, although he was a member of youth collective Young Bosnia and now was working under the patronage of the Black Hand, Princip longed for a better life for all the Balkan peoples.

Suddenly, he heard an explosion further down the street. Dust and smoke billowed into the air along with the screams of bystanders. His chest puffed out, eyes wide with a touch of pride on his lips. *We did it,* he thought. *We've assassinated the Archduke for all the Slavic peoples.* But before he could indulge himself further, the motorcade approached at speed. There, alive and well in his seat was Franz Ferdinand and although he reached for his pistol, Princip knew that it was already too late to shoot. His chance was gone, and he stood, watching the procession as it headed off toward City Hall, disheartened and ashamed of his inability to act.

Inside the motor car, Archduke Franz Ferdinand clutched his wife Sophie's hand. *What a terrifying ordeal this must have been for her*. Mother to his three beautiful children, it was rare for him to bring his life's love on such a trip. Having married well below his station, the Archduke was all but disavowed by his disgruntled family, and Sophie – petty nobility by birth and former lady in waiting to the heiress Ferdinand was meant to marry – was ostracized from official duties, often forced to enter a room last in keeping with her rank or not included at all. This rare treat of accompanying her husband had been enabled only by the fact he was in Bosnia on military rather than state business. Social class had no place here. Proud of his wife and his choice to marry for love, the Archduke wanted her to experience the pomp and ceremony from which she had otherwise been excluded. Even now, after the narrow miss from the grenade thrown directly at his vehicle, he remained calm and focused, convinced that the would-be assassin Čabrinović, who was at this moment being pulled from the river and arrested after his cyanide failed to work, was just a lone madman.

The men in the car behind him had taken the full force of the grenade, and the Archduke resolved to visit them at the hospital where they were taken for treatment. Despite concerns raised by his head of security, he demanded the motorcade take them there after the planned visit to City Hall – but promised to leave the city swiftly afterwards.

Back on Appel Quay, the commotion had died down. People milled about the streets, talking animatedly about what they had and hadn't seen. Papers danced on a light wind in the gutter. Princip, unable to see any of his comrades in arms, turned behind him on to Franz Joseph Street. There, the well-known Moritz Schiller delicatessen was already busy with locals queuing for mid-morning treats. Princip lingered outside, breathing in the delicious aromas, and considered what he should do next. It was unlikely the Archduke's planned route would go ahead. His military guard had no doubt already begun evacuation via a secret route. Perhaps he should find Ilić? Perhaps he should just go home. But if ... if the Archduke were to continue on ... then this would be the perfect spot to wait. And the Archduke was known to be pig headed and brazen. Just then Princip's deep thoughts were distracted by a passing friend, keen to talk about the events of the day.

Back in his car, the Archduke checked his watch. It was 10.45am, *plenty of time to visit the hospital before we need to leave*. Suddenly, his driver turned sharply to the right off Appel Quay and down Franz Joseph Street. He heard the governor of Bosnia, General Oscar Potiorek, call out that this was the wrong way, that it was part of their original – now

x

abandoned – route and they would need to turn back. The car stalled, stopping sharply right outside Schiller's.

Hearing the commotion behind him, Princip turned, eyes wide. The Archduke was right in from of him, just feet away, and as his guard scrabbled to push the car back up the street Princip drew his gun. *Sophie, she's in the car*, he thought, hesitating momentarily. But his heritage weighed heavy on his trigger finger and, determined not to let this second chance pass him by, he raised his weapon and fired two shots. Both Sophie and Ferdinand recoiled, fell back, Sophie slumping with her head in her husband's knees. *Sophie, Sophie don't die. Stay alive for our children*, whispered the Archduke as blood spilled from his neck, soaking his military attire. Within minutes both were gone.

Back on the street Princip gasped. He didn't feel that rush of pride, the glory he had momentarily experienced less than an hour ago. Panic rose inside him as people on the street moved his way. There was no time for cyanide, he realized and desperately he turned his gun toward himself – but the weapon was knocked from his hands as the guards pushed him to the ground, arresting him for murder.

Although the average person in the Empire seemed little affected by the Archduke's death, the political ramifications were huge. Political alliances across Europe, ostensibly designed to prevent war, resulted in a speedy spread of hostilities. Diplomacy between the Austro-Hungarian Empire and the state of Serbia who were blamed for the assassination quickly failed, the flames fanned by France and Russia.[2] When Austria-Hungary invaded Serbia on 28 July 1914, Russia was already mobilized to support her Serbian kin. Germany were obliged – and by many accounts seemed eager[3] –to support the Austro-Hungarian war effort by treaty. A French alliance with Russia resulted in Germany marching on France via Belgium, giving Britain a reason to get involved in the fray. Within weeks, Japan jumped in, courtesy of an alliance with Britain, and by October, Turkey had leant her support to Germany. The following year Italy, despite an alliance with Austria-Hungary and Germany, entered the proceedings alongside the Allies, and in 1917 the USA also joined on the side of the Allies after Germany sank several American vessels.

In his cell, deprived of visitors and reading material, Princip listened for any scrap of news about the war. Too young to hang, he had been sentenced to 20 years in Terezin – a fortress that was later used as a concentration camp by the Nazis. He passed the days in disbelief that his actions had led to this. He had been just a boy with an idealistic dream, a unified Slavic state free from oppressors like Austria. Reports of the millions of deaths on the battlefields ate away at him inside, while tuberculosis ate away at his outsides, covering him with sores and forcing the amputation of an arm. His dreams of a united Yugoslavia crushed, he waited eagerly for the anonymity of death which finally came to him in April 1918. He had no idea that many would remember him as a radicalized Serbian nationalist hell bent on chaos, or that in 80 years' time, the impoverished citizens of Bosnia, reduced by civil war, would visit his grave in droves, not to hold vigil but to defecate in the absence of a public latrine.

Princip sparked a bloody conflict, but the conflict itself ushered in something far more dangerous, enabled by the poverty and movement of war. On the second Monday of March 1918, just a month before Princip's death, the world changed forever. A seemingly harmless cold morphed into a global pandemic that would wipe out almost five per cent of the world's population – and ultimately assist the Allied forces to put an end to the Great War. Commonly known as 'Spanish flu' in Europe, this outbreak proved to be far more deadly than the conflict itself, yet it has faded into history, a footnote to the devastation of the First World War.

Perhaps it is difficult now, after a century of bloodshed that has included the Second World War, the Vietnam War, the Falklands conflict, various hostilities in the Middle East and the back-stabbing brutality of the Cold War to imagine how oppressive the scale and viciousness of the combat between 1914-18 felt to those who lived it. It was described as a 'war to end all wars' by US President Woodrow Wilson, and according to his friend Colonel House, he feared 'the war would throw the world back three or four centuries.'[4]

After four years of fighting on the European stage, when no one imagined the situation could become more dire, Spanish flu emerged suddenly, a dark and mysterious force which made brief, localized cameos across the globe before striking quickly on a huge scale and wiping out 50-100 million people in a matter of months, 'the greatest tidal wave of death since the Black Death, perhaps in the whole of human history'.[5] In the confusion of war, deaths are misattributed, patterns of disease movement missed, and it wasn't until they were boots deep in the pandemic, mobilized by the sudden and unprecedented global movement experienced during those years of conflict, that contemporaries really began to see the full horror of what was happening before them. Even then, they didn't see the beast until it was upon them. Suppression of information to protect the war effort, barriers to communication across enemy lines and the slower speed at which people and news travelled at that time all served to keep the virus masked, and authorities on the back foot.

Then, as quickly as she came, she was gone, leaving humanity 5 per cent lighter and an empty space a global war used to occupy. But there was no time for licking wounds. Cities needed to be rebuilt, alliances re-meshed. Sharp focus was placed on what went wrong politically and Spanish flu became the ghost in the night, a scary story to make children wash their hands and say their prayers before bed. Slipping away under the shadow of the post-war rebuild, much of the history of Spanish flu became informal, oral, stories passed down generations. It wasn't until the end of the twentieth century, when the horrors of SARS and bird flu filled the public with apocalyptic thoughts that a wider gaze was cast across the analysis – the virologists, anthropologists and political commentators finally began to look for a whole narrative.

In each chapter of this book we will meet one person, or a community of people, and tell their experience of Spanish flu. We will see its impact on society, politics and public health as it moved across the globe, how it was managed and explained. We will meet Spanish flu face to face, and by the end each of those singular experiences we will have woven not just that bigger picture, but the legacy it has left humanity for the future.

PART 1

THE SECOND MONDAY IN MARCH

ORIGIN THEORIES AND THE TRAIL LEFT BY DISEASE

Chapter 1

Circling Patient Zero

Lying on his bed in the barracks at Camp Funston, Kansas, Albert Gitchell felt a bead of sweat trickle down his forehead. Pulling one aching arm across his face, the young private stifled a sneeze. All around him the men were sleeping, around one hundred and fifty packed together on wooden bunks in his dormitory alone, weary from their training, weary from the worries of war. Soon, most of these men would be leaving this camp, leaving the safety of the USA for the shores of France. There, they would battle the army of the Kaiser – and many, perhaps most – would not return.

In June 1917, Fort Riley in Kansas was selected to be the largest of sixteen divisional military training camps designed specifically to get drafted troops ready for the Great War in Europe which the USA had recently joined. Construction had commenced in July, and Camp Funston was officially opened on 1 December 1917. Designed like a city, 15,000 carpenters built between 2,880-4,000 buildings that would accommodate over 40,000 soldiers. With its own pool hall, movie theatre, barber shops, restaurants, fire department, hospitals and police force, it was a huge achievement. The recruits were considered well-cared for before they were deployed east on their mission to bring down the central powers of Austria-Hungary and Germany, fighting alongside the British, French and Russians in terrible conditions very far from home. It seemed only right they should be afforded some small comforts before they departed.

By March 1918, the Great War had already killed millions of soldiers and civilians across Europe. This 'war to end all wars' had raged across Europe for four years with no real end in sight. Young Gitchell considered that as a mess cook, he might be one of the lucky ones – he might go on to live a little, have a family, perhaps tell his grandchildren stories of this terrible time. Stories of the men he shared space with at Funston, of the dusty summers and the icy winters, the hopes and dreams of those who didn't return …

Gitchell felt a chill run down his spine. In a moment of weakness, he turned his aching neck and tried to focus on his bunk-mates in the dark. It must have been about 4am and he'd had a fitful sleep. In spite of the fact it was only about ten degrees outside, Gitchell was burning up, suffocating in the heat his body was generating. Boiling in his own sweat, he had spent most of the night trying not to cough and sneeze and wake the other men up. They wouldn't thank him for that.

He'd had a cold for a few days, nothing serious. There seemed to be a bit of it going around. Some of the lads had 'visitors' the previous weekend, a few of the officers had strayed into town … You know, these bugs, they aren't hard to pick up. But this one, for Gitchell at least, kept hanging around. Just last night as he served what passed in the mess for a Sunday dinner to the other lads, he'd felt an ache in his shoulders, deep in his bones, that he knew wouldn't be resolved by a night on a lumpy mattress.

As the sun threatened to rise on the morning of 11 March Gitchell struggled out of bed. It took him twice as long to put on his fatigues as usual, due to the uncharacteristic weakness in his limbs and troubling double vision. He gagged at the thought of cooking breakfast for hundreds of men. Finally, he stumbled out of the barracks and instead of reporting for duty in the mess, arrived at Hospital Building 91, where the duty medic recorded a fever of over 103°F – more than 39°C.

Dizzy, Gitchell heard the medic's voice far away telling him that, just as a precaution, he'd be put in the contagious diseases ward. Telling him not to worry, the camp surgeon would be there soon and he'd be fine. He felt hands on his shoulders, settling him back against a comfortable bed. Gitchell felt his body being moved, gently wheeled to a different room, voices and faces swimming around him, distant, not quite in tune. Almost delusional, Gitchell allowed himself to sink into the mattress, thankful for the chance to rest. He blinked twice and watched the hazy figure of the medic hurry away.

In a different part of Camp Funston, Corporal Lee Drake was struggling to get his breakfast down. A truck driver assigned to the Headquarters Transportation Detachment's First Battalion, Drake wondered how he could be expected to drive when he could barely focus on his coffee. Heaving himself up from the bench, he staggered to report for duty, hot and bewildered. When his Sergeant told him to get down to the hospital wing, Drake didn't protest.

The medic was surprised to see another man arrive with identical symptoms so soon after Gitchell himself. He placed Drake in the same ward and when Sergeant Adolph Hurby turned up with a temperature of

104°F shortly after, he sent immediately for chief nurse, Lieutenant Elizabeth Harding. *It's not uncommon*, Harding thought to herself as she walked from bed to bed, *for sudden outbreaks like this to occur. After all, these young men are living in such close quarters, and many are from such remote farms they may not have been exposed to many contagious diseases before.* But as patient after patient came rolling in that morning, she realized that something quite unusual was going on. By the time her superior, Colonel Edward Schreiner, arrived around noon, over one hundred men had been admitted.

Schreiner was a meticulous and sober individual[1] who wasn't prone to panic or fancy, but when he arrived by motorcycle at the hospital, he knew straight away what he was looking at was serious. As he examined each man, recording similar temperature and symptoms, more came in presenting the same way. This was an outbreak, a contagion, and he arranged to send word to other camps so precautions could be taken.

Over the next five weeks, Gitchell's virus infected around 1,100 men at Funston, more than could be accommodated in the infirmary, and Schreiner requisitioned a hangar as temporary ward. Although Schreiner was relieved in many ways that only 48 of those patients died, this death toll was still high considering these men were young and fit. The rest of the patients, after a short stay in the infirmary, were shipped off to France to take part in the war, many still coughing and sneezing as they stormed the beaches. And yet it came as a surprise that by May 1918, reports of this virulent and mysterious virus had spread across Europe, wiping out legions of soldiers and civilians alike.

Gitchell was lucky in some ways. He wasn't one of the 48 at least. He went on to live a quiet life with wife Emma, but not being blessed with children,[2] those war stories rarely got much air time. It was after his death in 1968 that he gained immortality by being patient zero in most people's minds. In reality, he was simply the first recorded case. Medics offering origin theories as early as winter 1918 eschewed the idea that American soil could harbour any responsibility. Their fingers pointed to France and to China, but part of the reason they struggled to identify where the outbreak came from was because they didn't know what it was. In 1918, the idea of the virus was exceptionally new.

The word influenza was first used in Italy in 1504, when an unusual alignment of the stars was seen as the 'influence' of an epidemic. Various pandemics swept Europe in medieval times, but as the way symptoms were recorded was ad hoc and varied according to the beliefs localized communities held about disease, it can be hard to pin down their cause and categorize them by modern standards. Miasma theory, the idea that 'bad air', usually the result of rotting organic matter, was responsible for outbreaks such as plague, was strongly held, alongside ideas about astrology and spirits. In 1557, documented evidence of disease across Europe suggests a possible flu pandemic. A violent malady that swept Europe, Asia and Africa in 1580 was most likely influenza. The term influenza seems to have been first used in England around 1743, when an outbreak of fever and respiratory disease caused the death toll in London to treble, but it wasn't until the late 1700s that distinct features of the flu virus we know today were recorded and attributed as characteristics of a specific disease. That disease became a regular winter occurrence across Europe, with outbreaks causing death in those weakened by other conditions or age. Occasionally, history shows us a spike where young and healthy people were affected just as much, but smallpox continued to be the condition of greatest concern in the eighteenth century, with cholera taking over as the nineteenth century progressed.

In 1898, the term 'virus' – a Latin word meaning 'slimy liquid poison' – was used by Martinus Beijerinck to describe a pathogen smaller than bacteria that affected tobacco plants. A Dutch microbiologist and botanist, Beijerinck had successfully repeated the 1892 work of Russian botanist, Dmitry Ivanovsky. Ivanovsky had used a filtration system to remove bacteria from tobacco plants infected with tobacco mosaic disease, but noted the plants remained infectious afterward. This meant there had to be another cause than bacteria, one that at that time could not be seen – and which Beijerinck wrongly believed was liquid in nature. This idea was not new and had occupied scientific circles for some time. Even Louis Pasteur, one of the fathers of vaccination and proponent of germ theory (which slowly replaced outdated and incorrect ideas about miasma), had suspected some diseases like rabies were caused by something smaller than bacteria and therefore could not be seen under a microscope. In 1901, avian influenza, first described in 1878 and called 'fowl plague', was shown to be a virus by using the filtration method, but the link between avian flu and human flu wasn't to be made for another 54 years. This was in part because science already believed it had found the cause for flu.

Since 1892, the majority of the medical world had subscribed to the idea that human flu was the result of Pfeiffer's bacillus – a bacterium isolated by German bacteriologist Richard Pfeiffer from samples taken from the throats of flu patients. Pfeiffer was well respected, and a student of Robert Koch who had identified the specific bacterial causes of diseases like tuberculosis and cholera. Koch's methods had been applied by others to identify other bacteria with huge success, and Pfeiffer's bacillus garnered so much support that in 1918 it was used by the French and US governments, among others, to create vaccines. Support wasn't universal though, and critics noted that the bacterium wasn't found in all flu patients and was also found in healthy patients. William Park and Anna Williams of the New York City Health Department cultivated bacteria from the infected tissue of flu patients and found that not only was the bacteria Pfeiffer lent his name to not always present, but that when it was, it wasn't always the same strain – which would be very unusual in a pandemic.[3] But attempts to confirm the flu was a virus using filtration experiments had produced mixed results, and the vaccine seemed to be having some success, probably against secondary infections like pneumonia, reducing mortality risk. As a result, confusion and panic reigned, and as early as October 1918 military medics were pointing their fingers east.

Thousands of miles away in Imperial China, Dr Wu Lien-teh was working in Tianjin, on 19 December 1910, when an urgent telegram arrived informing him of an outbreak of disease in northwestern China. It was four years before the outbreak of the Great War and he was occupied training military doctors. Well respected, he was the first medical graduate of Chinese descent from Cambridge University in 1902 and had worked in Europe until recently. Now, it was he the Qing dynasty were calling upon to help rein in this terrible disease. China was still locked in dense tradition, with the average person turning to practitioners of ancient herbal medicine, suspicious of 'new' Western ideas around disease. The government requesting his European-trained eye demonstrated a huge shift in ideology. Wu knew it would be a difficult job, but to be asked for directly was such an honour! He made arrangements to travel right away.

Having decimated the border town of Manchouli, the disease was moving along the railway lines and public panic had set in. The ruling Qing dynasty was already on its last legs. The people of China – those in power at least – wanted change. It was essential that this outbreak was dealt with swiftly before it crossed the border into neighbouring Russia or travelled further south. It had already made it to the city of Harbin and there were reports of hundreds of deaths each day. Over 60,000 people would be killed in four months.

When Wu Lien-teh arrived in Harbin, he looked around him in disgust. Finding a handkerchief to cover his face, he picked his way gingerly through the filthy streets. In 1898, this had been a relatively small village but the establishment of the Chinese Eastern Railway had encouraged rapid growth. The result was a lack of infrastructure, poor living conditions and a migrant population speaking many languages and dialects. In addition, there was nothing really in the way of a public health strategy and victims were simply being quarantined in inhumane conditions more likely to encourage the spread of disease. There was no effective way to give information on prevention and care to the city's tightly packed residences and little interest from the authorities in the Western medicine Dr Wu knew was their only hope.

With the full force of imperial authority behind him, Dr Wu acted swiftly, suspending non-essential train travel and setting up plague hospitals and disinfection stations around the city. Supported by the police and military he imposed quarantine, which was unpopular with the people. Suspecting the public were hiding their sick and their dead, house-to-house searches became commonplace. It was brutal, he knew, but this disease was ravaging the people of China over a wide distance, and he needed to get the spread under control.

The symptoms patients were presenting with, such as coughing up blood and a purplish hue to the skin, made him suspect pneumonic plague early on. Trouble was, the only way to confirm that was to conduct a post-mortem – strictly prohibited under Imperial rule. Feeling bold, and sensing the ruling Qing's desperation, he applied for and was granted a dispensation. It was an historic moment, the first ever legal autopsy in China. As he cut carefully into the flesh of a recently deceased Japanese woman, the significance of his role was not lost on him. Gently and respectfully, he took the tissue samples and returned her body to a tidy state. After cultivating the bacteria, his conclusion was infection with *Yersinia Pestis*, a known cause of plague.

Now he knew the cause, his attention turned to the dead. The only hope of curtailing plague was to prevent exposure. There were over 2,000 unburied bodies at the city gates and come the spring thaw, the rats would probably act faster than the grave diggers, causing a boom for the disease. Dr Wu achieved a second, incredible dispensation, by convincing the authorities to cremate rather than bury victims – another major strike against Chinese tradition.

By April, the plague was all but gone and Dr Wu Lien-teh received another telegram – this time informing him he had been awarded the rank of major so he could be given an immediate audience with the imperial family.

Celebrated in all quarters, Wu went on to have an illustrious career which included laying the foundations for a public health system in China that would marry the Western medicine he had studied in England with Chinese traditions. The Qing dynasty barely saw another year, however, with revolution ousting them in favour of the People's Republic. In spite of Wu's high honours under the imperial regime, he was not a target during this coup and in 1917, when the people of Shansi began packing the hospitals with similar symptoms to those in 1910, Wu received another telegram.

On the surface of it, things in Shansi looked quite similar to Harbin, with symptoms such as chest pains, fever and coughing up blood. *This has to be plague*, Wu thought. *But why are so few people dead?* Plague is virulent and aggressive; at that time it usually killed quickly and regularly. Very few touched by plague lived to tell the tale. But while people in Shansi were dying, they were not dying in droves as they had in northwestern China seven years before. There were no piles of icy bodies at the city gates. A man of science, Dr Wu decided he needed to perform an autopsy. Perhaps bolstered by the permissions and successes he enjoyed before, he made no effort to seek permission from the relatives of the deceased before making his first incision, and the coach he was living in while in Shansi was surrounded by an angry mob and set alight. Terrified by this turn of events, and with a lack of cooperation from regional authorities around the need for quarantine, Dr Wu fled back to the capital of Peking (Beijing). Tissue sample in hand, he was convinced he had found plague present in the dead. But China had changed since the coup, and Wu was about to find out his views were unwelcome.

In the capital, he relayed his findings to the government. *The leaders in Shansi don't agree*, they told him. *They believe it is just a winter sickness, that it will pass.* Wu insisted. *We must instigate a quarantine*, he told them desperately. The disease had already spread by 500km, over 300 miles, in just six weeks. But the lack of corroborating evidence from British doctors also working in the region, the low death rate – only around 100 reported at the time – and the fact the people's republic wanted to remain strong, neutral and profit from the war resulted in a dismissal of Wu's concerns. Angry and worried, Wu decided to take matters into his own hands, and approached the press. Soon the newspapers were filled with reports that Wu had found plague. *Now the government will have to act*, Wu thought.

They did act, but perhaps not in the way Dr Wu anticipated. Two other Chinese doctors were invited to test Wu's samples, and neither found evidence of plague – the media reported the diagnosis was wrong, and none of Wu's recommendations were put in place, even though they would have succeeded in preventing the spread of this relatively mild, so far unidentified disease. The impact of this took its toll on Dr Wu, who had to be officially relieved of his duties after a bout of angina – although some suspect he was shuffled away due to an inability to tow the party line. [4]

The 'winter sickness' disappeared as suddenly in the spring of 1918 as it had arrived a few months before and became largely forgotten. After all, Russia had recently withdrawn from hostilities after their own revolution installed Lenin's new Marxist state and America had just joined on the side of the remaining British and French allies. After three and a half long years of fighting, the politicians, military strategists and the people of Europe felt 1918 was a turning point, that this would be the year the war would end, and there was no time to worry about respiratory disease in neutral China. Plus, the support of the People's Republic was essential. Since 1916, men had been secretly transported to France and Russia to work. Called the Chinese Labour Corps, their role was to support the military effort with heavy lifting, trench digging and maintenance, but they would never lift a weapon. After China declared war on Germany in August 1917, this activity was stepped up. Between 1917-18, 94,000 Chinese men were transported to the trenches, mostly via Canada in sealed train carriages (to prevent escape), before being loaded into the hold of ships, a journey that took around three weeks. Evidence of disease among these men was downplayed by authorities, partly because the importance of their role in the war effort meant a delay in shipping labour was unthinkable, and partly because of racism – Canadian doctors checking the men on route downplayed the symptoms of flu witnessed in some of the men, citing their 'inferior' or 'lazy' nature. After a quick rubber stamp, these men were then readily sent on to their final destination – France – where they came into contact with many British, American and French drafted troops.

Standing in the queue to enlist in the winter of 1915, 18-year-old Harry Underdown felt nervous. *I'm not exactly military material*, he thought, catching a glimpse of himself in the window. At just over five feet tall and about nine stone in weight, he knew he didn't look the part. But many of his friends, not much taller or heavier than him, had enlisted over the last year, and he knew it was the right thing to do. He was strong, having grown up on the family farm, Hodge End, and he could throw a hay bale several yards – he felt sure he could manage a gun. Approaching the counter, he pulled himself up to his full height, but the recruiter barely threw him a glance. He was male and of age and therefore was needed by his country, whatever his size. *Well done, son*, the recruiter barked, stamping his card with 'reserves'. *We'll call on your when we need you*, he said, and Harry was left to return to his relieved family at the farm.

In April 1916, Harry was busy helping his dad sow the fields when the letter arrived. He was to report to Surrey for training, and quietly he packed his bags and said his goodbyes. He felt excited but solemn. He was torn by the desire to serve his country and the tears beading at the corner of his mother's eyes. His parents had been hopeful that he may not be needed and as he walked down the path on to the quiet rural road than ran past their house, the promise he would be home soon still fresh on the air, they wondered if they would ever see him again.

Harry's time training at the army depot was marred by sickness. One bout of tonsillitis followed another and at one point he imagined he may well have served his country best back at Hodge End. Tired and weak, he watched as the men he arrived with were sent on to war, then another group, then another … Finally, in August, he was given the all clear and was shipped off to France with the rest. Standing in the trenches, the hot, dry sun pounding down as he wilted in his thick uniform and the sound of artillery fire ringing in his ears, he almost felt some nostalgia for the hospital ward in Surrey. Suddenly a shell exploded nearby, throwing him against his fellow men in arms, debris raining down until that hot sun was completely extinguished.

Shell shocked and with memory and speech loss, Private Underdown recuperated at a military hospital in Nottingham before volunteering to head back to France. It was February 1917 when he arrived back at the sprawling British military camp in Étaples. The Western Front was made up of around 440 miles of trenches, slicing the French landscape right up to the Swiss border. But the British troops arriving on the beaches of Northern France having crossed the slither of water we know as the Channel, were first squashed into the military camp purpose-built in the coastal town of Étaples – also a mustering point for the Chinese Labour Corps.

Right from the start, Harry could see it was a hellish place. A temporary home to around 100,000 men, many of them the sick and injured back from the Front, he felt he might prefer the bitter cold and constant rain of winter in the trenches to the stifling conditions he was forced to live in at the camp. He was, after all, an outdoor man, used to the isolation of the farm – not being hemmed in like cattle. As he made his way to his mustering station one thing stood out to him – the sound of sneezing. *It is winter*, he told himself, passing yet another man coughing into his filthy uniform. *Of course, some people would be sick.* But within a few days, he had heard about a terrible bug that was sweeping through the trenches, a bronchial pneumonia, the doctors were calling it, and a few days after that, Harry noticed a sore throat and a crackle in his chest. Two weeks after his arrival, he was sent to the hospital at Étaples with severe respiratory distress.

Lying in bed Harry clawed at his neck, unable to breathe. He felt his own eyes bulging in their sockets as he gasped for air. Reaching out, he clutched the edge of the bed weakly, swinging his legs across to try to stand. He struggled, his legs shaking. Gagging, he coughed some yellowish ooze into a pan at the side of the bed. *Private Underwood, you must lay down*, barked a nurse, but he could see the kindness in her eyes … the pity. A figure stood at the end of his bed, a doctor, listening to his ratchety breathing, seeing how his face turned purple with each failed gasp. His lungs filled with purulent pus, he struggled again to find his breath. Eyes wide with panic, he reached out, reached for the comfort of the nurse. Surely, she knows what to do with me, he thought, remembering the gentle way his mother had tended to him back home on the farm when he had been sick as child. But medical teams at Étaples were flummoxed. This mysterious and virulent disease had appeared suddenly on the Front and resisted all types of treatment. A common trait seemed to be the pus, and inability to breathe. Private Underwood died soon after this development, and 156 other men were carried off with him.

A study was undertaken by Lieutenant Hammond at Étaples and published in *The Lancet* in July 1917. This came to the attention of a team at Aldershot army barracks in England, who had their own outbreak of purulent bronchitis to deal with around the same time. Consultant physician at Étaples Sir John Rose Bradford, was perhaps the first to realize that what both camps were dealing with was the same disease. A whole eight to nine months before the mysterious respiratory disease appeared in Shanshi, China, it wasn't until the twenty-first century that researchers would ask themselves which direction it may have travelled in first.

Almost a year to the day after Private Underdown was gasping for his last breath in Étaples, Dr Loring Milner was on his way to see a patient in Haskell County, Kansas – just five hundred miles south from Fort Riley where Albert Gitchell was stationed as mess cook. February was usually cold, but this year had been particularly biting, and so Dr Milner had been called out to a few more patients than usual with what was known locally as 'knock me down fever'. When he got a call to say an older patient of his, a lady who lived on a remote farmstead, had the characteristic signs of the fever – chills, a high temperature and a ratchety cough – he knew he should attend immediately. Most people recovered from this bug, which he knew to be influenza, after a few days of bed rest, but the particularly old and young were vulnerable to complications.

Dr Milner had served this remote rural community for a long time and was well respected. He knew his patients personally and had a good memory for their varying medical histories. He ran a local drug store and people would come to him for a variety of advice. He treasured the people he looked after – not that he'd ever let on. Pulling up outside the farmhouse, he could see the lights ablaze. Before he'd even stepped out of the buggy, a young relative was guiding him urgently inside. He made his way upstairs and into a room where the entire family crowded around the bed. There his blood was turned cold by what he saw. The old lady, the matriarch of the family, lay helpless and struggling to breathe. With each rattle of her lungs she would violently cough up blood but remained unable to catch her breath. Although he struggled to carry out his usual examination, he identified the problem straight away. *It's pneumonia*, he told the family gently. *A secondary infection from influenza*. He administered opium for the pain, but there was little else he could do, and his patient passed away a few days later.

Her most terrible death troubled him greatly and not just because he had been unable to treat her. While secondary infections from knock me down fever in the elderly weren't uncommon, he had never seen such a violent presentation of symptoms. What he had seen, what the family had borne witness to, was truly terrible. For the next few days he turned the scene over in his head again and again, as he manned his pharmacy, wondering if there was something he missed. Before long, though, the old woman's death troubled him no longer. By the end of the week, he had had a dozen patients with the same symptoms and the list grew and grew. Even more troubling than the virulence of their disease were the patients themselves – young, strong and fit men and women who lived healthy and active lives on their farms. In just a few weeks, Dr Milner was called to treat 18 cases of influenza, with patients displaying similar symptoms to the old lady, many struggling to breathe. Thankfully, only three of them died. Between visits in his horse drawn buggy, Milner tried to find a pattern, an answer. In his exhausted state, he drew a vague connection – all the people who had been stricken seemed to work closely with animals. Was that important? He wasn't sure. The government didn't seem to think so. He wrote them a letter, urging further investigation, but it was mostly ignored, with just a one-line summary appearing in the public health reports in April – weeks after the outbreak at Camp Funston, where Haskell County local Ernest Elliot visited while his young son Mertin was sick. Another local, soldier Dean Nilson, was stationed at Camp Funston and came home on leave during Dr Milner's influenza crisis, returning back shortly before Gitchell reported sick.

It would be another twenty years before the medical profession even knew what a virus actually was and more than three decades before they made the connection between birds as incubators and animals as carriers, transmitting these lethal, mutated viruses to humans. The concept of acquired immunity and how populations are impacted by a new disease depends on their exposure to older varieties is still being untangled and where this particular strain originated from may never be fully understood. But deep in the throes of war, these early, poorly understood, often dismissed and largely unreported outbreaks of what could have been Spanish flu certainly hold significance, if not in understanding how it spread, certainly in ascertaining why it spread the way it did.

Chapter 2

Three Waves of Death

Standing in front of the medical officer, Private Harry Pressley tried to keep his head up and back straight the way the doughboys had been taught, but he felt like there was a crushing weight on his shoulders, pushing down into his chest. He was hot, even though it was early spring and the air still had an icy edge and he was tired, bone tired. *And you've felt like this for a couple of days you say?* asked the MO, listening to the crackle of Harry's chest. *Yes sir,* Harry wheezed, feeling a weakness in his legs. His nose was running but he didn't have a tissue. He thought momentarily of the way his mama would look after him when he was small, feeling his brow and bringing him ice water, or hot soup, when he was sick. *Well, looks like you're over the worst of it,* said the MO. *You work in the office, don't you? You'll be fine. Make yourself a hot drink for the sore throat.* And with that, Harry's appointment with the military doctor was over, and he struggled back across the drilling ground to his desk, legs like lead weights in the spring chill.

It was March 1918 and Pressley was working at Camp Dix in New Jersey, a training and staging camp for the American Expeditionary Forces (AEF) about to head off to Europe. Pressley himself wasn't going Europe, he was doing other vital work in the back office. But his mate, Cid Allen would be – at least if he was well enough. Pressley had seen Cid two days ago on the drill ground, as he ran an errand across the camp. Cid looked terrible, red faced with a hacking cough. The drill sergeant was yelling at him that he was too slow. All across Camp Dix, men had been coming down with this bug, and it had turned into pneumonia in many. Pressley knew what pneumonia looked liked and he knew he had the starting of it as well. But the collective war effort, he guessed, was more important than the individual man's health. *I'll manage,* he thought. *I'm only shuffling papers, and I'm out of the cold. Poor Cid though.* That night, at dinner, Pressley saw Cid in the corner, struggling to finish his meal. *You still sick?* he said, looking at his friend's fragile form. Cid Allen nodded sadly. *And they're shipping us out soon,* he sighed. *I've seen the doctor, but he just told me to keep drilling, there's a war on after all.* A few days later, Cid Allen along with the rest of the 15th Cavalry boarded their troop ships for the transatlantic crossing to France. Pressley was there to wave the men off. But during the crossing, a journey time of about a week, the bug swept the ship. By the time they reached Bordeaux, about 15 April, thirty-six men had fallen sick, and six had died. Many more would of course go on to perish on the battlefield, but Harry Pressley never found out which group his friend Cid Allen had belonged to.

Camp Funston may have been the first US military location that recorded the flu, but it wasn't an isolated incident. Within days of Gitchell's admission to hospital, men across a range of US military locations began coming down with the sickness, with many developing pneumonia. Colonel Schreiner, alarmed by the outbreak at Funston, had contacted colleagues and superiors across the country with regard to the speed and virulence of the virus among the men he'd seen. Soon, Major General Hugh Scott would be doing the same, taking up his concerns about the outbreak at Camp Dix with US Surgeon General William Crawford Gorgas even inviting him to come to Dix to check that they'd taken every precaution to stop the spread. Gorgas' response was to say that the pneumonia would abate if each man were given his own room – in other words, while the camps themselves might be clean, the nature of the conditions under which the army lived, sharing their living and sleeping spaces with large number of other people from across the country, was in itself creating conditions perfect for the virus. And yet still the army packed their soldiers, even the sick ones, into tiny, tight spaces on poorly ventilated ships and sent them to Europe.

One hundred years on, we still don't know where the Spanish flu started. The fact that there seem to have been so many simultaneous outbreaks across America with no obvious pathway for the spread, foreshadowed by the spectre of the unidentified 'winter sickness' in Shansi in late 1917, and the unexplained outbreaks of 'purulent bronchitis' in Étaples and Aldershot, determining the point of origin is rather like trying to complete a jigsaw puzzle with several missing pieces. What we do know is that the First World War was a major contributor in the development and spread of the virus. In order to explain why, we first need to find out a little bit more about the virus itself – we need to know what they didn't know in 1918.

We now understand that there are three different types of flu virus, A, B and C (with a recently proposed fourth subtype 'D' found in cows). It is type A that causes pandemics. There are several different varieties just of influenza type A, which can be found in humans, other mammals like pigs, and birds. In 1918, the medical profession knew flu was a specific disease based on its symptoms and clinical characteristics, but it wasn't until 1933, fifteen years after the Spanish flu outbreak, that it was confirmed that it was a virus, not Pfeiffer's Bacterium, that actually caused the disease. Once the electron microscope had been invented in the late 1930s, it became possible to see the virus – which was too small to be seen under a normal microscope – for the first time. In studying the structure of the virus, researchers were eventually able to see there were two different proteins on the surface – Haemagglutinin (H) and Neuraminidase (N). As time went on, scientists discovered that in each major flu outbreak these proteins are slightly different – each strain of flu is slightly different. Spanish flu is known as H1N1 while, for example, the Asian flu outbreak in China in 1957 is known as H2N2 and, the Hong Kong flu a decade later is H3N2. Finally, there is antigenic drift. This is the term for minor changes in the shape of the proteins in an already established strain. To put it another way, imagine influenza is a shop that sells only jumpers. Inside the shop, there are three main styles of jumper; V-neck, sweater or cardigan – these are the three main subtypes. Each of these three styles comes in a variety of different colours and sizes – and the shop stocks new colours and expands its range of sizes all the time. Once you have chosen your style of jumper, you select the size and decide on a colour – this is the strain. Once you've been wearing the jumper for a while, you might decide that you prefer it with the sleeves rolled up, or the buttons undone, or you find you've subconsciously unpicked the hem – this is antigenic drift. It's still the same style of jumper in the same colour and size, but it looks subtly different because of something that has happened over time.

It is this variability, the way the virus changes and adapts, that makes it tricky to fight. When a human gets a virus, the immune system tries to fight the virus off by first releasing protective chemicals called cytokines, followed by antibodies that attach themselves to the virus and destroy it. This battle of the tiny Titans causes the infected person to have a high temperature, body aches and feel generally terrible until the internal war is over. Most importantly, once your body has conquered the virus (as most do), it remembers it and, should you get it again, your body can send out exactly the right antibodies to knock it off quickly – less of a battle, more of a quick upper cut. This is how vaccines work, by exposing you to a tiny, controlled amount of a pathogen so your body knows exactly how to fight it later. When it comes to bacterial infections, this is spot on because they don't change, but viruses – presumably fans of Darwin – keep adapting to survive. A virus needs a host and if that host has a defence system based on recognition, then the only way to get past it is to don a disguise.

In spring 1918, the virus that swept across America, the battle fields of Europe, and began to spread to other countries via troop movements, was a new strain of flu – a brand new jumper in a size and colour not worn by humans before. In his book, *Flu Hunter*, international expert on the influenza virus Robert Webster explains that when two different influenza A virus strains infect the same cell, they mix their genetic material together to produce a new, hybrid strain of flu. This is called 'reassortment' and can result in up to 256 genetically different 'offspring' virus'. In the late 1960s, Webster, then a graduate student, and his friend Graeme Laver secured a grant of AUD500, (a substantial amount of money at the time), to study diseased Mutton Birds off the north-eastern coast of Australia. What started as, in his own words, 'a bit of a lark' kicked off over a decade of in-the-field research that established the now accepted fact that water birds, including ducks, are carriers of flu viruses. From the water birds, who largely remain unaffected by the virus, they spread to domestic animals such as poultry and pigs and from there can spread to humans. The process of reassortment as it passes from species to species creates a new virus to which the majority of the population – having not been exposed to before – has no immunity.

The 'mild' spring wave in 1918 did kill people, and it killed them in numbers in excess of the usual, seasonal flu – although this wasn't well reported due to censorship, and the fact that everyone was distracted by war. As usual, it was the very old and the very young who suffered high mortality from that first wave, which presented in what scientists call a classic 'U' shape – if the U is the line on a graph, then each tip represents the ends of the spectrum of population age, with the majority of people – those aged 15 to 60 – down the bottom in the low risk area, their immune system strong enough for the fight. However, between the end of the first wave that hit Europe and America around July/August 1918, and the start of the second wave in September, something happened which created a super strain, a more virulent virus than had ever been recorded. It has been suggested that antigenic drift caused a minor change to the strain with a major outcome – although it is almost unheard of for antigenic drift to occur so quickly, within a matter of months.[1] The virus that emerged in the second wave however was deadly, killing some victims within hours of exposure, and unlike most seasonal flu outbreaks, if you plot this one on a graph it has a distinct 'W' shape with a mortality spike in the middle of the age range spectrum – it seemed to be targeting victims aged 15 to 44.

By September it was apparent that Private Harry Pressley's war wasn't destined to be fought in the back office. As the Allies, with a little help from Spanish flu, managed to push the German line back, America mobilized more troops and young Pressley got his adventure in France after all. But on 11 September 1918, in Brest, he came down with flu. *Nothing more than the usual grippe*, he told himself, using the local name for influenza. *Nothing to worry about.* But over the next few days his slight fever and aching head became a burning temperature of about 30°C, with delirium and a constant struggle to breathe. As he lay in his hospital bed, barely conscious, he was aware of the nurses and orderlies working around him. *That new fellow will only last a couple of days*, he heard one say about him to another. *Keep him warm and comfortable as possible, that is all we can do.* Pressley lived to tell the tale (and write a memoir about it) but many other men did not.

The answer to the question of why some people escaped with their lives while others were condemned to a truly miserable death isn't fully understood and what has been pieced together is very complex. However, it has been suggested that part of the answer lies in previous exposure. Those who, like Pressley, suffered at the hands of the spring wave seemed less likely to succumb to the autumn outbreak. Another theory posited regarding the relative survival of the older generation, is that those who lived through the Russian flu of 1889-91 might have had some acquired immunity,[2] while very young children, still being breastfed, may have piggy backed off maternal immunity. While the question of the role of background immunity is tricky to answer, the importance the role a lack of immunity played is clear. As mobilized troops moved around the world, they took the virus to some of the most isolated communities on earth – and as a general rule, the more isolated people were, the harder they were hit. As we will see in upcoming chapters, the path cut by European troops through the various colonies was a path lined with death and those deaths were, by vast majority, of indigenous people, not those from the West.

The USS *Leviathan* left New York on 29 September 1918, carrying 1,000 men from the 57th Pioneer Infantry of Vermont, and 2,000 crew. They had already lost many troops on the journey from New Jersey, men dropping like flies on the march and the ferry crossing to NYC. Before she set sail,

120 men were removed from *Leviathan*, too sick to travel. Within 36 hours of setting sail to France, 700 men had come down with flu, and one man had died. The sick bay was full, leaving infected men confined to the tiny berths shared with many others. While the crew struggled to source 1,000 extra sick beds, those not showing symptoms were moved to a section of the ship that was so poorly ventilated it had previously been deemed unfit for human habitation. The official report of the crossing describes the horror on board; the pools of blood and vomit, the groans and terrified cries of those delirious with disease. The men were dying so quickly they couldn't be embalmed fast enough and were beginning to decompose on board; desperate, those in charge ordered the dead to be thrown into the icy waters of the Atlantic. Because the dog tags hadn't been issued yet and the patients had been too confused and ill to tell anyone their name, the identities of many of the bodies were unknown. According to historian John M Barry, when *Leviathan* arrived in Brest on 8 October 1918, 2,000 men were sick, and over 90 were known to have died.

The diaries of military chaplain Ed Clark tell a similar tale for the USS *President Grant*. Sailing just ahead of *Leviathan* on 22 September, Clark describes it as a 'ship of death', and tells how the men raved deliriously, eyes bulging, gasping for breath as they died. What witnesses found most perplexing was the speed at which the virus seemed to kill, and that many of those affected died a painful, terrifying death seemingly drowning in their own bodily fluids. This was not normal for flu, which wasn't usually fatal unless the patient became vulnerable to a secondary infection like pneumonia. As infected troops continued their movement around the globe, similar tales of sudden and extreme death among the young began to arise from the civilian population as well.

Ciro Vieira Da Cunha, a medical student in Rio de Janeiro, leaned against a wall bathed in evening light. He was waiting for a tram to take him home after a long day of study. *Excuse me, does the tram for Praia Vermelha stop here?* asked a man out of the blue. *Yes, it does*, Ciro nodded kindly, always polite and helpful. And with that, the man collapsed to the floor without warning. When Ciro checked, he was dead. Meanwhile, off duty tram driver Charles Lewis in Cape Town was boarding a tram to take him three miles to his parents' house in Sea Point. As the tram pulled away, he watched with horror as the conductor collapsed to the ground. A few minutes later, a passenger seated behind him also collapsed, and then another – both dead. A further three passengers collapsed and died as they made their way to

Sea Point, Lewis himself helping remove the bodies to be placed on the pavement for collection. Then, less than a mile from Lewis's stop, the tram screeched to a sudden halt. The driver was sprawled over the controls, dead. Lewis sat for a moment in the quiet carriage, the autumn evening sun casting long shadows, contemplating this bizarre situation. One thing he knew was that he was glad to be alive and with that he walked the rest of the way, grateful for the fresh air and solitude. In Budapest, sixteen-year-old maidservant Ilona Molnar complained of feeling a little unwell around lunchtime. The lady of the house flew into a panic – it was early October and there were already 100,000 cases of sickness across the city. She promptly told Ilona to go to her mother's house or the hospital and agreed to cover her expenses. Carrying a small bag with a few personal things, Ilona set off up the street. She considered perhaps the lady's reaction was a bit much. But as she walked, Ilona felt weaker, more unsteady, a bit unsure of where she should be going. Exhausted, she sat on a wooden bench on a street corner, still clutching her bag. By mid-afternoon, passers-by began to stop and stare – the girl's face was blue, eyes distant. Someone sent for an ambulance, but the hospital was so busy it was 8.30pm before a specialist ambulance arrived and found Ilona slumped to the ground, having suffocated to death.

The main characteristics of this second wave – the way it targeted the young and healthy and killed quickly leaving a bluish tinge to the face – have been homed in on by researchers in the decades since. They have concluded that it was the result of a 'cytokine storm' in the active immune systems of the young and healthy. This virus, when it invaded the body, triggered an immediate and overly enthusiastic flood of cytokine proteins which are designed to regulate the immune response. When too many immune cells flood the infection site it creates inflammation. If the major site of infection in a patient was their lungs, then they filled with fluid due to the inflammation, causing patients to drown in their own bodily fluids. Lung samples from Spanish flu victims also show them flooded with neutrophils. A tiny part of the complex immune system response, neutrophils are basically the direct killers, isolating and eating infection at the site, sacrificing themselves in the process. The excessive flood of neutrophils in otherwise healthy patients during the Spanish flu outbreak actually damaged the lung tissue, contributing to the blue-faced asphyxiation witnessed in 1918. The findings of one 2014 study by Summers et al, even suggested that the bigger the size of a victim's chest (and therefore lung capacity), the more vulnerable they were to the cytokine storm. The H1N1 virus wasn't just a lethal killer in its own right, it turned the body of the healthiest of victims on itself.

Another group who were particularly vulnerable to dying from Spanish flu were pregnant women. Women of childbearing age were already in the 'at-risk' group for the cytokine storm. But studies from the USA have shown that while mortality for women in general was 4.9 in every thousand, for pregnant women there was a slight, but still significant, increase to 5.7 in every thousand, with a 2005 study focused on women in Derbyshire showing that this group was twice as likely to develop pneumonic complications. Modern studies have shown that women in the latter stages of pregnancy are at particularly high risk of mortality from new strains of flu, and even seasonal flu can cause complications that warrant a stay in hospital. This could be because of the body's need to suppress the immune system while pregnant to prevent miscarriage, and because of the way lung capacity is reduced and blood circulation changes to accommodate the baby. According to a 2005 study by Cambridge University's Dr Alice Reid, during the pandemic, in the UK, the number of women who died while having miscarriages increased ten-fold due to infection with the flu virus. In the USA, still birth was the outcome for 26 per cent of pregnant women who came down with flu, and anecdotally it is said there were many more premature births, which could have resulted in long term health complications for many children of the flu generation. Across the globe, stories of vast swathes of orphans, of towns where every pregnant woman died, of families destroyed by disease are numerous and heartbreaking.

At the height of the second wave of the pandemic, rumours about its source began to spread. It behaved so differently from normal seasonal flu and there was so much confusion in the medical community, that rumours of chemical warfare were rife. The idea that Spanish flu was a manufactured agent designed to help the Central Powers win the war remains barren of supporting evidence – and as we will see later, if it were true, it backfired terribly, as Spanish flu could be considered to have given the Allies their much-needed edge over the Kaiser's forces. However, there were chemical agents used in warfare (against the ruling of The Hague Convention of 1907), such as phosgene and mustard gas, and while they are not lethal in themselves, they do have two properties that could have a relationship to Spanish flu. They damage the alveoli in the lungs, causing respiratory problems and increasing vulnerability to infection and they cause genes to mutate. It's possible that these chemical agents could have stimulated the virus to mutate in exposed soldiers, although it is a hypothesis impossible to confirm a century on. It can be seen from hospital reports that the men with flu who had been in a chemical attack suffered horrifically from bronchial and pneumonic complications, their lungs stripped and weakened by the gas then attacked by their own immune response. But at the height of the pandemic, there was no time for reflection. Few notes were taken, limited observations were recorded. Whether you came down with the disease or were supporting the infected, each day was a matter of survival, a list of basics that needed to be carried out just to make sure people were still breathing at the end of it. It wasn't until the second wave petered out just before Christmas that there was a chance for the global population to turn around, look back on the past few months, and let out a collective 'wow'. Even then, there were only moments to consider the enormity of it all. By January, the demobilization of troops that came with the armistice instigated a third wave which carried on in some parts of the planet until 1920. While it was by no means as impressive in its destructive power as the previous outbreak, it was still a killer knocking down people apparently in their prime.

In his 1919 report to the British Society of Medicine, Colonel A.B. Soltau made an observation regarding the virulence of the epidemic's second wave, which seems very astute considering that at the time, science still didn't even know what pathogen had caused the disease. Soltau noted that the 'law of redistribution' – the way military ranks are broken up and pieced back together during a high-energy offensive like that on the Western Front – could actually be a contributing factor to the spread and strength of epidemic diseases. In the case of Spanish flu, those men with some immunity were separated and put back together with men who had a different level of – or no – immunity. Some of the men were carriers, showing few symptoms but taking this deadly disease to those with no ability to fight it off. And although Soltau's report was specifically about the military, if you step back for a second and gaze at the passage of the epidemic through this particular lens, you can see Soltau's theory played out on a grand, global scale. Flu needs a host to survive. Without a good supply of hosts, it will burn itself out, adjusting and becoming a lower level pathogen, an irritation like other seasonal varieties. But in 1918, we gave this flu just what is needed – a constant supply of bodies, many with exceptionally low immunity, in which to infect, multiply and adapt in the deadliest way.

Between 1914 and 1919, more people travelled further than ever before. Farm boys from rural America took boats to France. Labourers from Eastern China travelled by train through Canada to Europe.

Almost one million British men donned fatigues and travelled to the Middle East. The German army marched through south-eastern Africa, while the French army mobilized in the north-west of that continent. Colonials, loyal to the Commonwealth, journeyed half way round the world from Australia and New Zealand to support their brothers in arms. And as it travelled, this war machine, it made contact with previously isolated tribes in central Africa, remote villages in Brazil, Alaskan fur traders who rarely saw anyone except the postman. The First World War may not have caused the virus in the way some people feared at the time. It wasn't a man-made chemical weapon. But the war did give the virus an almost endless supply of bodies, living in close quarters, many malnourished with already compromised immune systems, many just emotionally exhausted, and plenty who had never experienced a virus like this before. The result was a pandemic like no other recorded, a pandemic that killed more people in six months than the Black Death did in four years. A pandemic which dwarfed the sacrifices of lives during both world wars of the twentieth century and shaped the civilization we know today.

PART 2

EUROPE, AMERICA AND THE ALLIANCES OF WAR

THE EFFECT OF THE PANDEMIC ON THE COUNTRIES IN CONFLICT

Chapter 3

'In flew Enza'

How the European Allies were affected by flu

Running from room-to-room with a huge grin on her face, Rose Selfridge thought her heart would burst with joy. *It's perfect, just perfect*, she told her husband Harry Gordon Selfridge, the millionaire department store owner. *I couldn't think of anything better to give you*, he smiled. But Rose's gift wasn't a luxurious sailing boat or a beautiful home, as other wealthy women might have craved – it was a hospital in which US soldiers could convalesce in Dorset, where the American Selfridge family now lived.

Rose was an accomplished woman in her own right, having inherited some money and property from her American businessman father when he died. She had only been four years old and her memories of the astute but loving man she called father faded quickly. Instead, she resolved to put his money to good use. As well as broadening her own horizons through travel, Rose had indulged her passion for music by learning to play the harp and had even invested in property development in her home town of Chicago, commissioning forty-two villas and artists' cottages to be built carrying her name. Although she loved Europe and was a true Francophile, when they moved to London in 1911 to pursue Harry's dream of opening a London-based department store, she felt desperately homesick, especially when the war broke out and they felt threatened by Zeppelin raids and challenged by the hardships they witnessed around them. The move to Highcliffe Castle had helped – it felt much more familiar, much more like their beautiful home Harrose Hall on Lake Geneva in the US. She loved to walk the rose gardens at Harrose and had carefully cultivated over 2,000 different varieties of orchid while she also cultivated their children, Rosalie, Violette, Gordon and Beatrice. She had loved that home, loved her place in Chicago society. One of her favourite things was to put on a little recital where she might perform on the harp or invite other talented friends to sing or play to raise some money for one of the many charitable causes she embraced. The move to Highcliffe in 1916 had reminded her of those days and sparked a renewed interest in 'doing her bit' – which is why she and Rosalie had volunteered for the Red Cross, working at nearby Christchurch Hospital.

It was never enough though. As she pored over the daily papers, read letters from her friends back home about the American effort now they had joined the war, she worried that there was more they could do. They had the money after all, and she had the time now the children were grown. *And now my dear, you can help in the way you wanted to, offering our young boys the recovery time they deserve*, Harry beamed, as if reading Rose's mind. Rose took a deep breath. She needed another walk around to take it all in. The cricket pavilion which had gone unused for so long was now an office, kitchen and 'mess hall' – a familiar but comfortable dining room where the patients could share a meal. There were twelve, two-man 'huts' built from wood with a rubber curtain against each side so they could always choose to be in sunlight. There was a big common area with books, games and a gramophone, and finally a bathroom, and private quarters for an American officer in charge of discipline.

Over the next few months a constant stream of injured men kept Rose busy at the hospital, but by spring the new arrivals had more than just bullet wounds and injuries of war – many were arriving burdened with fever and a heavy chest and Rose, who was prone to pneumonia herself, was glad she could host them at the castle where the fresh sea air and beautiful views of the Dorset coastline were perhaps the best medicine. Rose was right of course, good ventilation and plenty of rest are still the best treatments for flu a century on. But for Rose, whose own health had always been a little shaky and who was prone to contracting respiratory disease, having the men there was no help at all. At the start of May when she felt the fever come on, of course she took the doctor's advice of plenty of fluids and took to her bed. But a few days later flu turned into pneumonia, and on 12 May 1918, Rose died.

Harry Gordon Selfridge, always devoted to Rose (despite being seen on more than one occasion with another pretty young thing on his arm in London) was devastated. Meticulously, he planned her funeral and burial at St Marks Church, opposite Highcliffe, himself. Seamstresses from Selfridges embroidered a silk sheet with hundreds of red roses, and the men from the hospital who were well enough formed a guard of honour for the woman who had cared for them. In the wake of Rose's death, her husband kept himself busy, but Selfridge was never quite the same. Always a showman, he continued to spend extravagantly on mistresses and friends until the fortune he had amassed was all but gone, and he died comparatively penniless in Putney aged eighty-nine – ironically, also of pneumonia.

In May 1918, the war was not going well for the Allied forces. Germany had made gains quite far into France and the word on the street was that they were going to win. With Russia pulling out of battle after the Revolution in November 1917, the Kaiser had been able to concentrate his efforts on the Western Front where British and French troops were already weakened. More than a few prayers of thanks were said for the arrival of the American Expeditionary Force in April, although, they seem to have brought with them a respiratory disease that was knocking down as many troops as they could replace. Among the constant stream of injured men that were shipped back across the channel to convalesce at home were those who also had a fever, a cough, a streaming nose … With the men who came home to Britain arrived Spanish flu.

It is unclear where its main port of entry might have been but it didn't matter anyway. As the men spread out, via the railways, across the country to their loved ones at home, so the flu spread and took hold far and wide. In late May, the Glaswegian slums of Govan and Gorbals were paralyzed by a sudden epidemic that lasted eight weeks. Although this first wave was mild in comparison and most recovered, there were early deaths among those vulnerable to complications like Rose Selfridge. Eight children at an orphanage in Lanarkshire died between 18 and 28 May from influenza, with at least one succumbing just a few hours after symptoms began. The week of 19 May, a week after Rose died, has been suggested as the week the pandemic could be considered to have officially started in Britain, with 511 recorded deaths compared to just 79 the week before.[1] But the week of 29 June has been chosen, retrospectively, as the official date as it was the first week that the number of deaths of those under fifty-five officially outweighed those deaths of people over fifty-five[2] – a characteristic of Spanish flu that separates it out from the usual, seasonal variety.

The main impact during the first wave from May to August, though, was on the functioning of the country due to the number of sick rather than the number of dead. After four years of the ravages of war, food and fuel shortages were rife. People were malnourished and struggling to get by and were vulnerable to infections like flu. Morale was low with pretty much everyone in the country affected by the injury, death or disappearance of a solider on the Front. The more people who came down with the disease, which could put them to bed for up to two weeks, the slower the country became until it was struggling to function at all. By July 1918, *The Times* reported that some of the coal mines in Newcastle had as many as 70 per cent of their workers off sick, bringing production during a time of great need practically to a standstill. At the start of August, it was reported the coalfields in Wigan had a third of their men off. In the school yards, children were skipping to a new rhyme:

> 'I had a little bird,
> Its name was Enza.
> I opened up the window,
> And in – flew – enza.'

With wartime censorship attenuating the coverage of the outbreak in the UK, the name 'Spanish flu' was adopted off the back of reported outbreaks in Madrid and the fever of King Alfonso of Spain. *The Times* even suggested 'the dry and windy' weather, which they referred to as a 'Spanish spring' was to blame, and a good dose of British rain might see the disease off for good. No one was too worried (except perhaps those immediately affected), and while the mines and factories of the north were all but closed, the theatres and music halls of London were full – an upturn in Allied fortunes in France during June and July had also sparked an upturn in mood, and by the end of August reports of Spanish flu also petered out. The general feeling was that flu was over – and soon the war would be over too.

Sitting in his office at the Lister Institute, a young man whose name (not rank) was Major Greenwood, sat wringing his hands in frustration. Reports of flu, sporadic anyway during the first wave, had disappeared from the papers – and daily life – completely and Britain was carrying on as if that was it, over and done with. But he knew better than most, because he had science on his side. A gifted mathematician who later trained as a doctor at Whitechapel hospital, Greenwood had been working as a statistician at the Lister Institute when the outbreak occurred. Plotting a graph comparing case data for the spring outbreak against the Russian flu of 1889-90, Greenwood saw a trend in the numbers that offered a chilling prediction – a second outbreak was on the horizon for autumn 1918 and it was going to be much, much worse. His fears garnered little interest from the War Office though, and a letter to General Medical Council representative and

Army Sanitary Committee representative Sir Arthur Newsholme was met with derision – it was more important, felt Newsholme, to keep the country moving and facilitate the war effort than to worry about flu. By the time Walter Fletcher, secretary of the Medical Research Council, who shared Greenwood's concerns wrote to *The Lancet* and the *British Medical Journal* in August urging preparation for the epidemic-to-come, the trenches of the Western Front were already rife with the second wave of disease. With the focus on the mobilization of the army, the very British need to 'carry on' and a refusal from local government to make concessions such as restricting travel by public transport or closing theatres, it was only a matter of time before it infiltrated civilian life again.

Gripping the steering wheel, Dr Sidney Snell wiped the sweat from his brow. To say he felt terrible was the understatement of the decade, but his phone had been ringing off the hook all morning, he had patients to see. The village of Christchurch was perched on the edge of New Forest, in Hampshire, an area of outstanding natural beauty that housed a tight knit community. Snell knew each of his patients by name, their likes, foibles and their family history by heart. Starting the engine, he knew he really should be in bed, but it was the middle of October and these flu cases had been building again for the last two weeks. With no other local doctor, he had to see this last patient – then he could rest. He took it slowly, driving down the bumpy country road with care in his relatively new automobile. But ahead of him was a curious sight – two donkeys standing to attention side by side like sentinels at each edge of the road. Whatever next! Carefully, he tried to negotiate the gap between them, but before he realized what was happening there was a terrible thump and the car came to a sudden stop. Clutching the door, he hauled himself up to survey the scene. There was only one donkey, positioned squarely in the middle of the lane, and he'd knocked it flat.

It was perhaps for the best that Snell killed the donkey, for it made him realize that he couldn't work with double vision and he returned promptly home to his bed. In other parts of the country, however, rural doctors became the vector for the spread of the disease. Acting as doctor, dispensing pharmacy and sometimes even performing minor surgeries, they were often the only accessible help for miles. But most inevitably came down with flu and under pressure to keep working, passed it on to those who may otherwise have escaped. In the Shetland Islands for example, Dr Harry Pearson Taylor was laid up in bed, his temperature almost 39°C when a local

woman was brought to him after having been hit by a car – he found her
dead on the floor next to his bed in the morning. In the cities, the picture
was no better, with hospitals becoming centres for the spread of disease.
In spite of the protestations of doctors such as Leonard Hill at the London
Hospital's Medical School that patients should have access to cool, dry and
fresh air – sleeping outside if necessary – the wards were slow to catch on
and many windows remained sealed, hospital furnaces burning hard in the
dead of winter, offering flu the perfect climate to multiply and infect. In fact,
some statistics even appear to show that those in the makeshift hospitals,
especially tent hospitals, fared better than their counterparts on the wards.
Data has since shown you were up to 40 per cent more likely to die from
flu in Britain if you lived in town.[3] This statistic is, in some ways, a bit of a
curiosity, as in other places – as we shall see – living rural was more or less
a death sentence.

By the end of October 1918, concern regarding the outbreak was so
high that it was raised in parliament. Across the nation, daily activities were
drawing to a halt, with bus and train services postponed, post offices and
bakeries on limited hours due to staff shortages and undertakers turning
down orders as they were already struggling to process the number of
dead.[4] In January 1919, during its annual meeting, the Prudential insurance
company noted that between 2 November and 31 December 1918, £650,000
was paid out to cover industrial losses from flu against £279,000 in losses
from war in the same period. In London, 1,500 police officers failed to
turn up for work which meant a third of the entire force was off sick. Once
infected with Spanish flu, those vulnerable to the heliotrope cyanosis
could be dead in less than a day. Older patients might suffer longer, finally
succumbing to pneumonia. In spite of all this, when the Armistice was
declared on 11 November, people lined the streets in celebration and in
Trafalgar Square, thousands gathered, waving flags and hugging strangers,
undoubtedly spreading the disease as statistics show the death toll peaking
shortly after.

As Joseph Wilson trudged down Carisbrook Street in Harpurhey, Manchester,
his bag was heavy and his boots felt tight. It was mid-November and very
cold. He watched as his breath condensed in the air before him, like the
smoke from heavy artillery just after it had fired. Not that he has seen much
artillery fire. As a member of the Army Pay Corps, he did a valuable job
fighting the Kaiser via finance. The men on the Front needed to be paid after
all! A music hall pianist and encyclopedia salesmen, he was never going to

be Front line material, but he was happy to serve his country from the back office – he just wished he didn't have to be away for so long at a time. It was cold, but the grey November skies of Manchester and sprawling brick tenements were a welcome sight. He couldn't wait to get home to his wife, Elizabeth, his daughter, Muriel, who was eight, and his son John who was just eighteen months old.

Arriving at number 91 he knocked gingerly, smiling. Then he knocked a bit harder but still no one came. Frowning now, he wrestled his key from his heavy bag and turned the lock in the door. *Elizabeth?* he called. *Are you home, dear?* From upstairs, he could hear the sound of laughter. Not like in the music hall, just a gentle, babbling chuckle. *Oh John*, he smiled. *Elizabeth must be playing with you. Perhaps Muriel has gone down the street to get something from the shop.* Joseph dashed up the stairs to his small family but turning into the bedroom he stopped in the doorway, paralyzed by the sight before him. There, sprawled out on the bed was Elizabeth, just thirty years old, blue and rigid, eyes staring lifelessly toward him. In her arms was Muriel, her face swollen, body bloated having died several days before her mother. And there was John, in his cot, no doubt hungry but smiling nonetheless, just happy to be in a room with his whole family, although it would be the last time.

John was raised by his maternal aunt until his father remarried, but he always felt that his father resented him for surviving his mother and sister during the pandemic. By the time his father died, John Wilson was at university and known to most as Anthony Burgess. He would become the acclaimed author of *A Clockwork Orange* and other dystopian works of fiction influenced not in small part by the death of his mother and sister and the childhood he felt he had lost.

There are many stories of lost childhood from the pandemic. The number of orphans in England, Scotland and Wales increased sharply as a result of Spanish flu, although there is little in the way of official statistics. Up until 1918, adoption was a very informal affair, an agreement between private parties, while churches and charitable organizations ran orphanages for the poor children who couldn't be homed elsewhere. However, it is telling that in 1918 three philanthropic organizations were founded, the National Child Adoption Association (NCAA), founded by Clara Andrew; the National Adoption Society (NAS); and the National Council for the Unmarried Mother and her Child (NCUMC) to deal specifically with this issue of rehoming children, in which the state would have no formal involvement until later into the 1920s. There were many who children failed to gain life during 1918. There were 2,500 deaths of pregnant women, [5] which in reality, constitutes the death of 5,000 people even though the unborn children weren't officially recorded in this way. As N.P.A.S. Johnson has pointed out in his paper on the topic, it would also have prevented an untold number of future births from taking place. Research has shown the mortality of women aged twenty-five to thirty was 600 times higher in 1918 than in the previous four years, and pregnant women had a fifty per cent higher chance of developing pneumonic complications. The year of 1918 was also the first on record where the number of deaths outweighed the number of births.

During the official 46 weeks of the pandemic in England, Wales and Scotland, the Registrar General recorded over 170,000 deaths. These figures only account for deaths from influenza and its immediate and recognizable complications – there are many more, no doubt who could be added to that list, and it has been suggested by commentators that the real death toll could be closer to 220,000. Most of those who died were aged 15-44, and it appeared to hit all social classes fairly evenly – crowded living conditions and poor sanitation did not seem to make it much more likely that you would die. A third wave, again mild but still responsible for several thousand deaths, arrived in early 1919, further exhausting Britain's limited supply of medical staff and supplies, and the country's tolerance for tragedy.

In Paris in November 1918, French poet, Blaise Cendrars, walked slowly behind the procession taking the body of his friend Guillaume Apollinaire from the Church of St Thomas Aquinas to Père Lachaise cemetery. His head hung in sadness as he thought of his wonderful friend, aged just thirty-eight, who had achieved so much already. An acclaimed poet and a war hero, it was unthinkable his life had been cut short by this terrible affliction. He smiled dryly at the irony of it – *Guillaume survived the trenches, taking shrapnel to the head, and now he had been carried off by something as trivial as flu* ... He wondered if his friend, the man credited with creating the term 'surrealist' would appreciate the bizarre twist his life took at the end. But he could ponder no more, because ahead there was a huge commotion. It was a celebration for the Armistice, called just days after his friend had expired, Apollinaire may well have heard the anti-Kaiser shouts of á mort Guillaume! Death to Wilhelm! from his own deathbed, and now the mourners were forced to walk through the laughing, kissing crowds who were singing ironically, 'No you don't have to go Guillaume!'.[6]

Since April 1918, Spanish flu had been quietly creeping across France, working its way from the western ports and the Front toward the north. But on the ground, the average person may not have noticed. The initial wave was so mild, with barely any excess deaths registered in the statistics at all. In the trenches, although many French soldiers came down with flu, very few deaths were recorded. It wasn't until September, when the second wave set in, that civilians began to notice. Spain closed their border with France at the end of September, and by the middle of October, in Paris, deaths due to the pandemic had reached around 4,000, with almost 8,000 Parisians recorded as dying from influenza over the course of the year.

It's perhaps no surprise that it took a while for the hysteria in pedestrian France to build. The French Armed Forces were a tidy bunch, who as a result of good discipline around sanitary measures had more or less eradicated all the usual contagious diseases that waged wars within the men fighting wars, such as typhus, dysentery and smallpox. In the towns and cities though, no such discipline existed. A neglect of public health services, coupled with unhealthy cultural norms like spitting, on top of wartime hardship, meant that outbreaks of communicable disease were rife nationwide. While the milder form of influenza had been rumbling through the troops for months, many other parts of France didn't even see the virus until the second wave started in September, and statistically speaking, you were 40 per cent more likely to die from the virus if you lived in an area that had not been invaded. In addition to the increased mortality rate for those not exposed to the weaker form was the tendency for the virus to affect people aged 20-40 more heavily – a trend that was retrospectively named 'Apollinaire's syndrome' after our poet. Women were also more susceptible. While it was noted during the epidemic that in Paris rich and poor prefectures were attacked similarly, with some of the richer areas having a higher death rate, it was later revealed that many of these statistics related to female servants, aged 20-30, living in cramped and often squalid conditions in the attics of the bourgeois houses where they served.

With 80 per cent of the French medical profession attending to men on the front line, and local councils paralyzed due to a lack of direction or any centralized approach to health from the government, the way in which the epidemic was approached varied greatly across the regions. The result, however, didn't seem to matter. In Marseille, the local council did nothing, while in Lyons they did a lot – but their death rate was more or less the same. In Bordeaux, burials, rubbish collection and the supply of water all came to a standstill after men and horses were requisitioned for the front line. In many city hospitals, they had to erect camp beds on the wards to take more patients, and the lack of isolation contributed to the spread. The Ministry of the Interior, the Public Health Council and the Académie de Médecin all ordered the closure of theatres, cinemas, markets and churches in the autumn – but on the ground this was not enforced due to a lack of manpower.

Although by Christmas infection and mortality rates had dropped considerably, a third wave was yet to hit the country. Peaking in February 1919, it caused a further 2,270 deaths in Paris[7] just as the peace process was starting. Although we often talk of the Great War lasting four years, 1919 is the often unacknowledged 'fifth year' of war, when, although the fighting in the trenches had been halted, fighting around the political table was just getting started. After years of bloodshed, fragile land gains, revolutions and abdications, each delegate arrived in Paris with a set of demands – and those delegates were not immune to flu. As we will see in chapter 11, it is possible that Spanish Influenza had a marked effect on the outcome of the war once the documents were finalized in April 1919.

The biggest civilian legacy of Spanish flu in France and Britain, however, was the foundation stone it laid for a true public health system. Until 1918, post-Darwinian concepts of Eugenics had been growing in popularity, but the way in which Spanish flu swept across Europe made policy makers think twice about where blame should be laid for illness. Having insurance systems to pay for medical care wasn't enough – in fact those systems not only collapsed under the weight of a crisis like Spanish flu, it could be argued they actually contributed to the severity of the problem by alienating those who often needed care the most. The focus on health as being the responsibility of the private individual also took the onus away from state to provide citizens with crucial medical advice, to ensure the availability of doctors, nurses and drugs and to provide an organized strategy to combat mass infection. It was time to place the responsibility for healthcare squarely on the state and although those systems took some time to develop during the twentieth century they had their roots in Spanish flu.

Russia was the first to put such a system in place in 1920. While they had withdrawn from the war in 1917, they had been suffering the hardships of revolution and civil war alongside Spanish flu in 1918 and early 1919, brought home to them from the Front by released Russian prisoners of war. Their healthcare system, developed under the watchful eye of Lenin, was put in place as a result of his observations around the abject suffering of the working classes at that time and the growing disciplines of biometrics and epidemiology played a huge part in Russia's vision for the health care of the future. They realized that in order to keep large populations safe from epidemics, you needed to look at infection trends across those populations, not just treat each individual who presented with symptoms.

Perhaps because Russia did it first, the concept was slow to gain popularity in other areas. In Britain, we didn't benefit from a full National Health Service until after the Second World War, in 1948, in part because of its apparent relationship with socialism (of which many politicians were very suspicious). However, changes to the National Insurance Act of 1911 meant that by 1936, half the adult population had affordable access to modern hospitals and GP care, including lower paid manual workers. Many GPs also created subscription services aimed at the middle classes who couldn't access the NI scheme, where registered patients paid a small weekly fee in exchange for using the service when they needed to. One such business, Pioneer Health Services in Peckham, London, was a forerunner to our modern health clubs. Opening its doors in 1926, it combined medical care with fitness facilities, such as a swimming pool, and a healthy cafeteria and promoted a holistic approach to fighting disease. Hospitals, previously funded by philanthropists and offering patchy care that was often based on social judgements, now became free to all with a small, universal weekly-workers' contribution used for funding. After the abolition of the Poor Law in 1929, many workhouse infirmaries became general hospitals. Many other buildings no longer needed outside of the poor law were adapted for other needs, such as to offer maternity services and many clinics offering free care for women and children sprang up nationwide.

France had long been a European centre for good medical practice, with the Montpelier university founded in 1289. In the nineteenth century in Paris, physicians lobbied for better hospital facilities, structured teaching and better sanitation and public health measures. By the Great War though, medicine was largely a private affair, available to those who could afford it with little focus on health and medical care of the general populace. Physicians were largely left to their own devices. The toll of war and the Spanish flu epidemic opened the eyes and minds of those in power, however, and in 1928, France launched its own system of national health insurance. Over the next seventy years, the government expanded the system to cover all residents and with no deductibles and generous coverage of costs, it was named by the WHO as the best public healthcare system in the world in the year 2000. Paris was also the home of the International Office of

Public Hygiene, an umbrella organization for twenty-three European states. Set up in 1907, it had largely been a collector and distributor of information, but in 1919 it expanded to Vienna and with the support of the Red Cross opened up an office dedicated to fighting epidemics. Later, after the Second World War, the then defunct Paris based organization, its American counterpart and the League of Nations would morph together to become the World Health Organization we know today. Many of the privileges of good health we enjoy in Western Europe were founded, and then built upon, as a result of the impact of Spanish flu on a population who until that point had largely been responsible for accessing their own medical care.

Chapter 4

The Naples Soldier

Flu and class divisions in the neutral territories

One tiny hand clutched inside her mother's firm grasp, María Dolores Vergés skipped light-footed along the beach. She loved these walks with her mother. Together they lived in the small town of Arenys de Mar, just forty kilometres, about twenty-five miles, outside the city of Barcelona and while it was a simple life, it was well loved. Six-year-old María shared a small house with her mother, father and brother, while another older brother lived with close family elsewhere in the town. Over the last few months, María had watched her mother's gentle physique swell, had experienced those beach walks getting slower and had seen the way her father had rested his hand on her mother's rounded stomach – soon, María would have a little baby brother or sister to play with. *I hope it's a girl*, she thought, imagining how she would share her toys with a little sister, and help brush her hair. *I can't wait*.

Arenys de Mar was a small town, a close-knit community, perched on the edge of the Mediterranean Sea. Each day, the fisherman would leave the port early and head out to find their catch. In the afternoons, after school, María and her mother would often walk to the harbour to see the boats come in and watch the daily fish auction before taking a stroll along the broad, yellow sands and dipping their toes in the warm sea. On Saturday mornings, María would help her mother at the market, buying their food for the week. She would trail behind, carrying heavy string bags as her mother strode home through the white washed two storey buildings of the town. By far María's favourite time though, were the village festivals in honour of Saint Zenzo in July, and Saint Roch in August, when the whole town would gather in the main square after Mass and enjoy folk dancing and food from street stalls, like freshly baked bread with sliced tomatoes, little parcels of salted cod or *buñuelos* – deep fried pastry dipped in sugar.

María knew there was a war on, and she knew that Spain was not involved. Other than that, the hostilities to the far north affected her very little. As she had sat, eating a portion of fish at the Saint Roch festival just weeks ago, she had listened to some older men speaking about how the festival used to be, food so abundant that some stalls would give it away for free to the little children. Although it was neutral, Spain had been hit by a lack of supplies due to war and hunger was more common than it used to be in villages like Arenys de Mar – the price of fish higher, there was more reliance on locally grown crops. But María did not remember life before there was a war and she did not know what it was like to have a never-ending bread basket. As long as she had her *buñuelos* and her mama, to her everything was just fine.

One thing María had noticed about the recent festival, though, was the people coughing and sneezing. That seemed rather odd for the summer. But then, her mama had told her about 'The Naples Soldier', this funny bug to the east in Madrid that had made King Alfonso so very sick. She hadn't said much more, though when at the festival María had sat next to a young man in his twenties with a terrible cough her mother had called her away quickly. *I'm tired, my darling,* she had said, pointing to her bump. *Perhaps we should go home early today.* María was sad, as she loved these celebrations, but she knew she had to be a big girl and make sure her mama got time to relax. Her father had told her so.

Since the festival, many people in town had been sick. María heard her father telling her mother late at night when they thought she was asleep. She had even heard her mother suggest she have time off school. *No, no, it will be fine I am sure*, her father said reassuringly. *The schools are still open, and you need your rest in the day*. A few times after school, instead of going for their walk, María had gone with her mother to check on friends and relatives who were ill, to make sure they had enough bread and milk and to see if they needed the doctor. Then one afternoon, it wasn't mama who picked María up from school, but her brother. *Mama is sick*, he told her gently. *She needs to rest for the baby*. The next morning, María gathered the string bags for the market, but Mama did not move from her bed. María went and sat beside her, putting one hand on her arm. An onshore breeze was blowing through the open window, cool and refreshing, but her mama's skin was red hot and clammy with sweat. *I'll go to the market with you today*, said her father, smiling in the doorway. But he looked strange and María knew he was worried.

Days went by and mama did not move from her sick bed. Each afternoon a different person would collect her from school and María would look longingly toward the beach, desperately hoping that tomorrow mama would be well and life could get back to normal. Her father was sick now and her brother too. She hadn't seen her older brother for a while. Back home, feeling dizzy and suddenly cold, she crawled into bed next to her mama and looked over at her pale white face. Her eyes flickered open and she smiled at María briefly, arm resting across her huge bump. María stretched out a finger and touched her mother's belly. *Not long now*, she whispered, before falling into a deep sleep.

María Dolores Vergés never met her baby brother or sister. When she awoke from her own flu-induced stupor, her mother and the unborn baby had died; her father and brother died a few days later. María's older brother came to fetch her when he recovered from his own infection and took her to live with him at the house of some distant relatives. For María, the experience was devastating – turning her whole world, her daily life and her expectations for the future on their head. Spanish flu took away her most treasured possessions, her family, and she was left alone and frightened as a small child to watch and wonder if she would be next. In a letter to historian Richard Collier, many years later, she recounted not just the devastation she felt, but how it reverberated through the whole village as each and every expectant mother with flu died, many taking other members of their family with them. She signed the letter, heartbreakingly, 'one who cannot forget'.

In other European countries, the course of many people's lives had already been changed irrevocably by war and influenza – devastating as it was – was just another tragedy to be factored into the 1,500 days of misfortune the people had already lived through. But in neutral Spain, the tendrils of war had so far only really made themselves known through scarcity of food, and even then, only in the lower echelons of society. The outbreak of flu was felt as a new, sudden and wholly more tangible danger to the Spanish, who also felt isolated in their experience as no country at war would admit to having it. Even as late as the end of June, the Spanish Health Department had received no official information about a flu epidemic in other European countries.

In 1918, Spain as a nation was experiencing a period of prosperity, brought about by the fact it wasn't involved in the all-consuming war. However, this also meant rapid price inflation which affected the working classes most acutely. As the machine of industrialization, still new in Spain before the war, got into full swing, and increased food prices left the agricultural workers – at the time, two-thirds of the Spanish workforce – wanting, people began to move in unprecedented numbers to the cities, and also to France, to find better paid and more reliable work. There is little doubt the pandemic arrived from France – even at the time this much was obvious. During the first three months of 1918, almost 25,000 Spanish workers migrated to France to replace the workforce that had been conscripted and sent to the Front, while 9,000 came back the other way. Without those migrant workers, the mutually reliant machines of both life and war would have ground to a halt in Europe. Travelling by rail, workers heading home from France would by and large arrive in Madrid, before continuing their journey outward to the provinces.

The first reports of flu in Spain hit the press on 22 May. Madrid-based newspaper *ABC* ran a story about a mysterious illness that had been sweeping the city, the spread encouraged by the region's annual festivals where more gatherings than were usual were experienced. Although the disease was very sudden, with rather alarming reports of people falling over from fever while walking in the streets, most people were not concerned. Just as in other countries, influenza came and went each year and while it was usually associated with the winter, summer outbreaks were not unheard of. In Spain, the spring and summer were full of local and national celebrations, *la fiesta*, from the now infamous *la Tomatina*, to localized gatherings celebrating obscure saints and regional harvests, the perfect vector for spreading a virus such as flu.

When the first cases were reported, most of Madrid was humming a catchy little number called 'The Soldier of Naples' from the operetta *The Song of Forgetting*. Even those not fortunate enough to have visited the opera recently were enamoured by the song, leading one newspaper to remark that this flu-like virus was just as catchy – and so in Spain the Naples Soldier is how the disease became known. In the rest of Europe though, where wartime censorship prevented the reporting of illness in the press, stories of the outbreak in Spain became popular news items and it wasn't long before the name 'Spanish flu' had been almost universally adopted.

A week after the *ABC* story, it was reported King Alfonso XIII had fallen ill, and after him the prime minister and several cabinet members. The disease began radiating out, reaching most parts of the country and Portugal by mid-June. The newspapers were full of stories from the various regions and towns, particularly central and southern Spain which were most affected but, by and large, the mortality rate was low. By July, it very much seemed to have all blown over and the average Spaniard was back to worrying about the price of bread. In late August, however, reports from the eastern coast between Barcelona and Valencia showed that flu was back and this time it appeared to be much more serious.

Authorities honed-in on the railways, understanding from the earlier outbreak the important role it played in spreading the disease. In early September, travellers from France were put under quarantine in Irun on the Basque border while inspection hubs were set up inland to try and control the spread. Portuguese workers were not allowed to disembark their trains at all until they reached their home station, which in at least one case meant a wait of seven to eight hours in a crowded, hot and unventilated carriage at Madrid. The sea ports, only very lightly used at this point, imposed a complete quarantine.

At the same time as authorities had their eyes on cross-border travel, Spain was erupting in localized festivities to celebrate the end of summer and the harvest. Groups of people gathered in ballrooms, theatres and town squares, packed in tight in joyous celebration. Many of these people had travelled from neighbouring towns or had been working elsewhere in Spain and were heading home – and they were not put under the same scrutiny as people crossing the border.

In the town of Valladolid in central Spain, 200 kilometres or 125 miles north of Madrid, chief health inspector Dr Garcia Duran had a difficult decision on his hands. Since the Feast of St Antolin in the first week of September, the outbreak of flu had been fierce. He knew that its spread had exploded after various gatherings around the small villages in the province. He had even been critical of the small town of Olmedo, that had agreed to press on with their scheduled bullfight even though every house in the town had at least one person sick and many deaths had already occurred. However, the town council had been worried about the cost – the actual economic cost – of not continuing with the event. And now Duran was left facing the same question. Should the city of Valladolid cancel its autumn festivities for fear of the spread of flu? It made sense to in so many ways, the death toll was already high and doctors were confused, unsure of what it was they were dealing with. In some regions, whole towns were at a standstill with no one to deliver mail or work in the factories. Panic was setting in. However, Spain's economic crisis had only got worse during the course of 2018. The gap between rich and poor was bigger than ever and Duran knew many were relying on this festival for income, perhaps to keep them going through the winter. Eventually he was persuaded; he would delay the announcement of an epidemic until after the festival had finished, because the economics seemed more vital than public health concerns. This was a scene that played out across Spain, and no doubt led to many more deaths.

The severe shortage of medical professionals in rural areas also contributed to fatalities. With no good advice to fall back on and no professional help to turn to, people were unaware of how to prevent the spread or make the afflicted more comfortable. Medical students from Madrid were sent to some rural areas, where they often found the sick in an unventilated room, friends and family gathered around, with alcohol used as a drug for comfort. Even where medical advice was readily available it was often conflicting, with a variety of treatments being offered from bleeding to diphtheria antitoxin. A strong reliance on Catholicism also aggravated the spread, with church attendance increasing despite the advice to stop public gatherings; some churches organized additional events to help cleanse the population of their sins – the suggested cause of the pestilence. After a week-long series of religious events in honour of the Virgin Mary, the spread of the disease in the town of Zamora was rapid, and they suffered the highest death-rate in any major city in Spain.

During October, while the epidemic was at its peak, almost 8,000 people died in Spain. Many newspapers used five pages or more for obituaries and the Church had to suspend the usual two to three days of prayers for the dead so infected bodies could be buried quickly. With just over 160,000 dying in total during the three outbreaks which finally ceased in June 1919, October 1918 accounts for more than 50 per cent of the Spanish deaths. Those areas that had a more comprehensive first wave in the summer had a lower death toll during the second and weak third wave due to acquired immunity and northern Spain did, in general, suffer a higher death toll than elsewhere for reasons that cannot be completely explained.[1]

In early September 1918, 12-year-old Karl Karlsson stood outside his home and watched the second coffin of the day be taken to the local cemetery. The central Swedish town of Österund was almost 600 kilometres, 370 miles, north of the capital Stockholm, nestled on the edge of the Storsjön lake. A centre for trade, they had suffered a hard war, even for a city so far away from the Front in a country that – apparently – wasn't involved. However, the blockade of the German coastline had severely impacted shipping to Sweden as well and food was scarce. The local garrison, on high alert in case the Swedes needed to choose a side, had caused the remote town's population to increase by 4,000 people, to 13,000, and they were struggling to cope. They didn't have the infrastructure for all these people – they didn't even have a hospital.

Just over a year before, when the sudden arrival of hundreds of labourers to start work on rail connections north had caused a massive food shortage, young Karl had watched in awe as both workers and soldiers rose up against the terrible conditions and poor rations, striking, protesting and disobeying direct orders. Some of the clashes with the authorities were quite violent and his father muttered that they'd never seen the like of it up here. In town, Karl knew, some people were living in terrible conditions – whole families in one room with nowhere to cook or wash. And the local Sami people weren't even allowed proper homes, they still had to live in tents by law. But where Karl's family lived on the edge of the town it was quite quiet. Except for the funerals of course. Since the Spanish flu had reached them several weeks ago, there had been several burials a day. He watched the quiet procession heading off down the road and shivered. It was unseasonably cold, and through the mist of his own breath he saw a few snowflakes fall gently from the autumn sky.

Spanish flu had trickled in to Sweden from Germany and neighbouring Norway – also neutral – since late June, but it wasn't until the ship *Torsten* made port in Gothenburg from London in mid-July that the epidemic really hit. It had boarded trains with workers, soldiers and even tourists and spread out across the country. By late August, the death toll in Österund was around twenty people a day with no organized government response and the city's Bank Director Carl Lignell knew something had to be done. He took funds from Stockholm through the banking system without authority and turned a school into a makeshift hospital. Even the local newspaper began organizing help, publishing calls for donations and offering up its offices to store supplies. Volunteers working door-to-door discovered something that may not have otherwise been revealed were it not for Spanish flu – the sheer poverty many of the people were living in just metres from the wealthy town centre where business and tourism boomed.

In Uppsala in the south of the country, the outbreak peaked in November when a record 5,000 cases were recorded in just one month – 30 per cent of the total number of infections in the region during the entire epidemic and the hospital was choked with influenza patients who made up almost 80 per cent of admissions. Patients were treated with cognac, camphor injections and wrapping in bed linen soaked in cold water to try and get them to sweat. In some cases heroin was used to reduce the violent coughing. Later it was discovered that not only were these treatments useless, they were sometimes harmful.

Initial advice from the Swedish Medical Board that the epidemic was 'mild in nature' delayed an organized response. Confused city authorities did what they thought was best for their area, with Gothenburg and Malmö closing schools in October, while in Stockholm they remained open. Although the military had been identified as both vulnerable to infection, due to their close quarters and potential spreaders, due to their cross-country travel and annual recruitment drive in September, military activity was not pulled back. Sweden was characterized at the time by a vast class divide and those at the lower end of the socio-economic spectrum were hit hardest by flu, as were the rural areas. In terms of public health, Sweden had one of the most forward-thinking systems having employed physicians to work in towns and regions since the 1700s. However, the medical board's delay in acknowledging the severity of the epidemic and the perceived need to keep military activities functioning made the country vulnerable, highlighting inequality in both medical care and standards of living which those in power had been able to turn a blind eye to for years.

The government was heavily criticized for the way they handled the pandemic, which peaked again in April 1919 and then again in the spring of 1920 – much later than in many other countries – with almost 40,000 people estimated to have died among the population of 5 million over the three years. Social unrest during the war and in the years after the flu outbreak directly informed change to the public healthcare system in Sweden over the next decade. The Hospitals Act 1928 made it mandatory for County Councils to provide inpatient hospital care for local residents, and by the 1940s, outpatient care – while still technically charged for as private – was fully refundable through the public system. In 1968, the National Board of Health and Welfare was formed and the structure of the current public health and welfare system Swedes enjoy today began to be laid. From the sparsity of services and draconian attitudes of the early twentieth century has grown one of the most egalitarian and efficient health systems in the world.

In May 1916, at 5am, a train arrived at the town Chateau d'Oex, Switzerland. The alpine resort had been deserted by tourists since the start of the conflict, the hotels empty and the mountains quiet, as it was difficult to reach neutral Switzerland across the fields of war. But today, 10,000 people stood waiting for the arrival of a very unusual set of visitors – just over 300 British troops who had been captured by the Germans and were officially Prisoners of War. Under a special agreement, Switzerland would be taking in wounded PoWs from all sides so medical staff could attend to their own men on the Front. With plenty of empty hotels in alpine villages to house the men it made sense and it also made Switzerland look useful and reduce the risk of them being invaded.

As the train rolled into the station, Captain Cyril Joliffe looked out of the window in surprise. As a PoW, he had been shunted from one German military hospital to the next. The conditions had been terrible and as yet, he had received no proper treatment for his wounded leg. When they'd all been marched on to the train, Captain Joliffe limping along on crutches, they had wondered what fresh hell they would find at the end of the line. Now, the people of the town were cheering as they arrived, throwing flowers at the carriages, *and was that … my goodness it was! A brass band playing!* Switzerland truly was another world from the horrors of war and he felt a tear wet his cheek. Later, as Captain Joliffe reclined in his bed having been seen by the doctor, he learned that not only would more men from all sides be joining them here, and in other alpine villages, but that his wife, Millicent, would be allowed to join him in a month or so as well.

Over the next two years, a total of 68,000 soldiers from France, Britain and Germany were accepted into Switzerland, some staying in villages and others at specially built camps. It was a pragmatic solution that probably sealed Switzerland's identity as a place of neutrality, perhaps even informing the choice of Geneva as the base for the League of Nations later on. Allowing PoWs and, in some cases their families, to live in the Alps reduced the threat of the war arriving on Switzerland's doorstep – but it did leave them vulnerable to a different type of invasion. By July 1918, flu had reached the PoW camps, either brought in by infected men or their guests. When the Swiss troops manning the border became sick, they were sent home – and the disease soon became prevalent throughout western Switzerland. By September, the second wave had taken hold of the whole country.

Men were much more likely than women to die in Switzerland with 60 per cent of the victims aged 20-40. The virus was violent, killing within hours in many places and incapacitating around half of the population. Just over 25,000 people died before the virus disappeared in January 1919, making Switzerland one of the hardest hit countries in Europe. Like Spain, it had not experienced casualties of war, and the public response was one of anger and frustration that this could have happened. On the ground, it was chaos, with schools closed but public transport still running; group gatherings in places like churches banned yet restaurants permitted to stay open. Local government and national government disagreed on what the best course of action was and misinformation was rife. With the army completely incapacitated by flu, the press launched an offensive of words against them, framing them as incompetent and demonizing Colonel Carl Hauser, the chief officer of the army medical corps. Press and public interest exposed how poorly prepared the Swiss Army was, without proper medicines or resources to tend to their seriously ill troops. The sense of public outrage was so strong that the government launched an inquiry which ultimately led to the reorganization of the army medical corps.

Meanwhile, as influenza reached its peak, a *Landesstreik* (general strike) was called by the politically left wing Olten Committee, which included Robert Grimm – an associate of Lenin. Around 250,000 workers laid down their tools on 12 November and some protested in the streets, bringing the whole country to a standstill for three days. The Olten Committee's list of demands included proportional representation in government, a 48-hour working week and pensions. As in Spain and Sweden, the outbreak of flu had revealed the huge class divide between those making a profit from their neutral war position and those who were suffering from the high inflation and food shortages. In addition, many families had been thrown into abject poverty after the men of age were conscripted into the unpaid Swiss Army to defend the borders, their families left starving at home. The strike was literally the 'haves' and the 'have nots' bearing down on each other. The government invoked the army to 'keep the peace' in response, bringing Switzerland to the edge of civil war. But after three men were killed by the army in Grenchen, the strike was called off and everyone returned to work. But the anger and resentment that had underpinned years of mild civil unrest in neutral Switzerland could not be put down so easily. Although 35,000 strikers were brought to court with prison sentences for Grimm and his associates, the changes they wanted slowly became a reality. In 1919, the 48-hour working week was introduced, with insurances for old age and dependants and votes for women coming along a bit later. Perhaps the biggest legacy for the Swiss was the change in the relationship between workers and employees, where the introduction of a system of collective bargaining and consensus-based decision making resulted in one of the most stable economies through the post-war period into the 1990s. Fearful of returning to the desperate times of November 1918, employers collectively agreed to institute the minimum wages and standards demanded by unions in exchange for assurances of cooperation from the workforce.[2] Some recession-inspired disruption in the 1990s notwithstanding, collective bargaining still underpins the Swiss industrial relations system today.

Chapter 5

School's Out in Vienna

The pandemic behind enemy lines

Crouched in a ravine, near the French town of Morcourt, Dominick Richert felt quite unwell. Perhaps it was to be expected. A non-commissioned officer in the German army, his company were positioned close to the Front and had been under attack from British planes and shells every night for weeks. On a rest day, not so long ago, he and three other men had crept through the thick fields of wheat to see what state the village was in. They had been horrified at the destruction. Most of the buildings were in ruins, with debris flung to the other side of the street. They found dead horses, bridles still tied securely to an uprooted pole and the bodies of soldiers in an abandoned wagon. Chilled to the bone, they turned and fled back to their company but barely escaped with their lives as British shells rained through the wheat fields around them. On another occasion, as he and a team returned from the Front to their company, they had to hide in a tunnel while the British stormed a nearby trench. They listened to the screams of their fellow countrymen as bayonets ran them through in the dark. Just a few days ago, they had watched as a British plane crashed near their hiding place. The flames from the fire were too strong for a rescue, but they dragged the charred corpse of the pilot out of the wreckage later and buried him nearby. Daily, the men in his regiment experienced things that would make any normal person sick to the stomach.

Richert hated this war. *I doubt anyone likes it*, he told himself, but he perhaps hated it more than most. Born in Alsace, a border region between France and Germany that had been hotly contested for as long as it had been inhabited, Richert identified to an extent with his family's French heritage even though his passport said *Deutschlander*. Viewed with suspicion by the German authorities, it was only recently that men from the region had been allowed to serve on the Western Front, so afraid were the German army of deserters. A decorated soldier with great skill in the field, Richert nonetheless viewed his role with enormous contempt. He constantly questioned authority and showed great sympathy for the soldiers they were charged to fight. *After all*, he thought, *they're just the same as me, here for the same reasons as me – because some high paid official told them to go.* Richert hated the politicians behind war, almost as much as the war itself.

Today though, in the heat of the July sun, he suspected his sickness was more than circumstantial. He had so far avoided the many infections and bugs travelling the trenches but, exhausted and underfed, he realized his body would easily succumb to whatever this sickness was. All around him, for the last few days, he had seen men taken ill. Pale, sweaty, vicious coughing and raucous sneezing – it wasn't just a common or garden cold, even he could see that but there was no sympathy from up top. Men serving at the Front were no longer allowed to be sick, only seriously wounded or dead. There was no time for any of that nonsense, he had been told, even though half the company had been struck down. Thankfully, he had been given a special job – to accompany an infantryman to Metz to pick up a deserter. It would take a few days and he was relieved to be getting away from the Front, especially if he had a bug.

It was somewhere between Rethel and Sedan, in a packed train carriage full of soldiers, that Richert felt the fever come on. One minute he was shivering cold, the next burning up, *and oh the thirst!* At the next station, he fought his way from the car and gulped down water from a drinking fountain. He knew he must have flu and, reading a newspaper, he realized it must be this Spanish flu which had broken out at the end of May. Quite a few people had died in Madrid, where the paper said it had started and he knew he needed to take his condition seriously. That night, when they arrived in Metz, they stayed at his companion's family home and he was thankful to take off his uniform and sleep in a bed – the first time in nine months. *Oh, how glorious this feels! Even with flu ...* After spending some time the next day looking around Metz, Richert went to the military canteen where he felt so awful that he gave his food to two Italian POWs charged with cleaning the plates. He had seen them earlier sneaking leftovers and felt sorry for them. The next day, Richert shivered on the train journey back to the Front, although he did manage to eat some fresh cherries he had purchased before boarding. Fruit had been hard to come by in his four years of service and even with flu they tasted like nectar. At the station before Cambrai, he was shocked to hear an announcement that everyone from his division should disembark. They had been relieved from duty at the Front and were holed up in the German-occupied village of Bévillers, such was the severity of their sickness.

Richert reported to the doctor for an examination – *if you could call it that*. After being asked what was wrong, the medic gave him a peppermint tablet and told him to go and make some tea. *How ridiculous!* He thought to himself, angry. *They may as well just tell me to go and die somewhere else!* Richert had been allocated quarters in the house of a French family and they were kind to him, despite being under German control. The daughter, who spoke a little German, explained his sickness to her mother who brought him a duvet and plenty of sugared tea and encouraged him to sweat his illness out. The occupied French villagers were sent food parcels from America – an agreement with the Germans – so they had sugar, cocoa, meat and bread which the family shared with Richert – he felt so grateful for their care. After two days, his company were given new orders but he was so weak he had to sit on the machine gun wagon while they marched. In Mars-la-Tour, close to the important Front at Verdun, a medic told Richert he would have to stay behind – he was far too sick with flu to go on. But the food was so terrible and the beds full of lice that after a few days he pretended to be well so he could be discharged. It was 35 kilometres, about 20 miles, to where his regiment were positioned and he only made it to his company because another kindly soldier let him ride an army horse. Too ill to fight, he spent six days lying flat on his back in a dugout while he recovered. *I can't go on like this,* he thought. *Four years of service and this is how they treat a sick man.* On 23 July, while in active service just a few hundred metres from the Allies, he and two others managed to escape across no-man's-land and defect to France as many other men from his region had done – a *déserteur Alsacien*.

Richert and his company were probably some of the last soldiers to fall victim to that first wave of flu in the Spring of 1918, which began sweeping the trenches on both sides around April and peaked in July. About this time, things had been looking rather dire for the Allied forces and Germany was feeling quite confident it could win this war. With Russia finally signing the Brest-Litovsk treaty on 3 March 1918, signalling the end of their involvement in hostilities, Germany was able to divert a myriad of troops and resources from the Eastern Front to fight France and Britain in Western Europe. More than one million men, along with several thousand pieces of heavy artillery, were sent west where the Germans out-numbered the Allied forces with a ratio of up to four to one

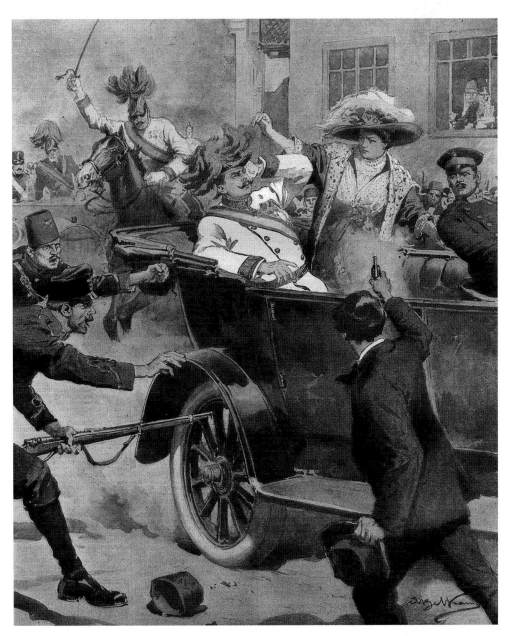

Archduke Ferdinand shot by Princip, by Achille Beltrame for Domenica del Corriere, 1914.

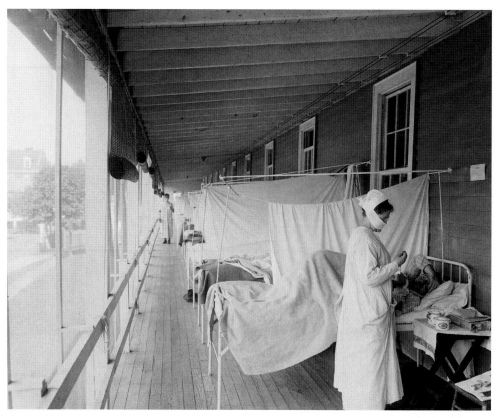

Walter Reed Hospital Flu Ward, Washington D.C., USA. (Harris & Ewing Photographers).

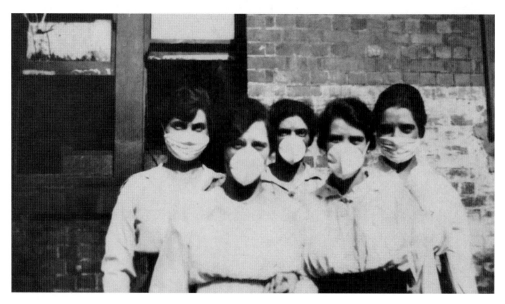

Women wearing surgical masks during the influenza epidemic, Brisbane, Australia, 1919. (John Oxley Library, State Library of Queensland).

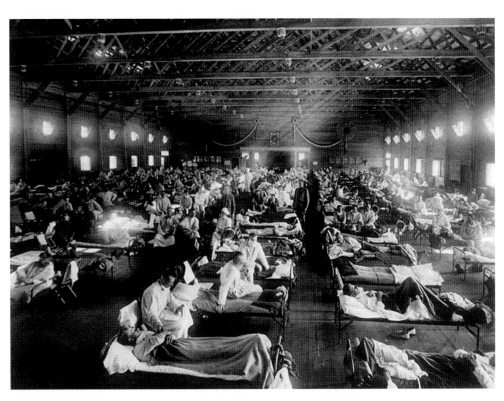

Emergency military hospital during the influenza epidemic, Camp Funston, United States. (Image courtesy of the National Museum of Health and Medicine, Armed Forces Institute of Pathology, Washington, D.C, USA).

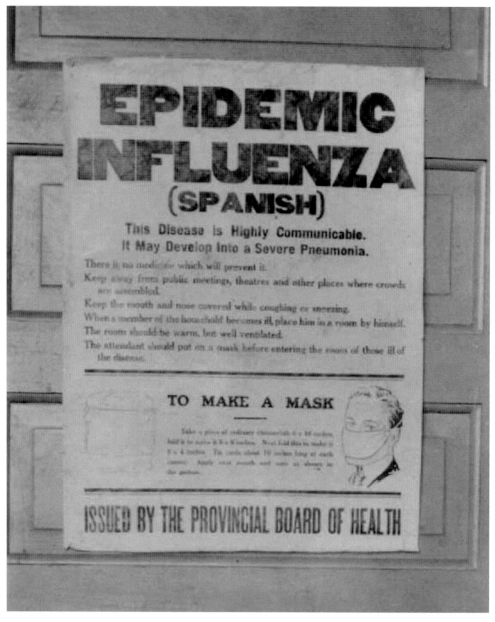

A poster issued by the provincial board of health in Alberta, Canada, alerting the public to the influenza epidemic, circa 1918. (Glenbow Museum).

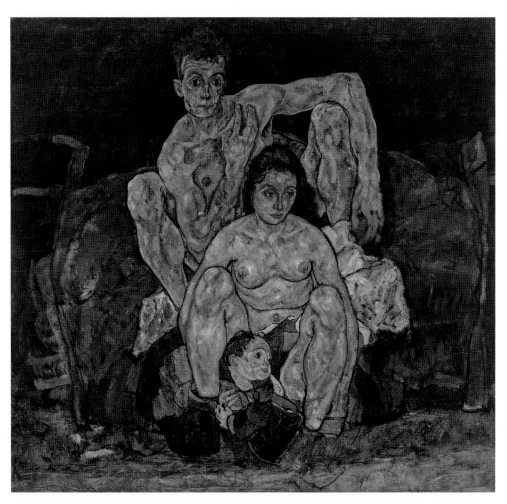

Egon Schiele, unfinished family portrait.

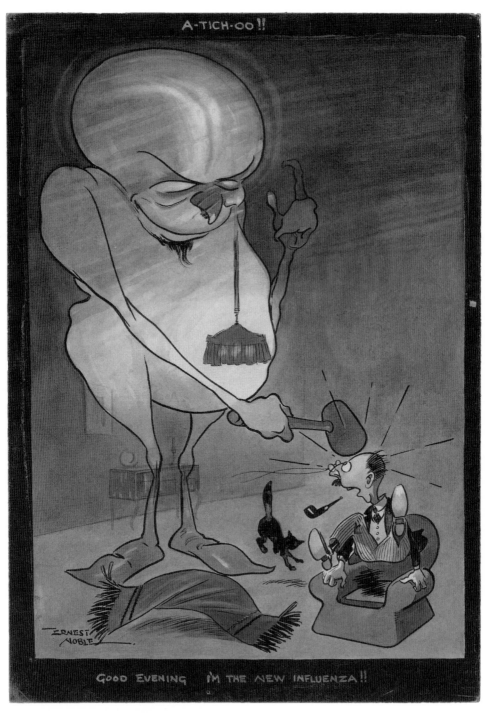

Good evening, I'm the new influenza! Cartoon by Ernest Noble circa 1918. (Wellcome Library)

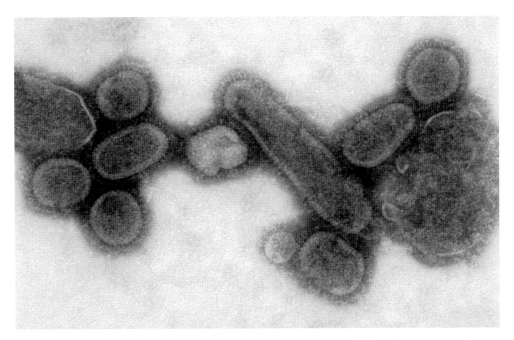

This negative stained transmission electron micrograph (TEM) shows recreated 1918 influenza virions that were collected from the supernatant of a 1918-infected Madin-Darby Canine Kidney (MDCK) cell culture 18 hours after infection. (CDC/ Dr. Terrence Tumpey/ Cynthia Goldsmith).

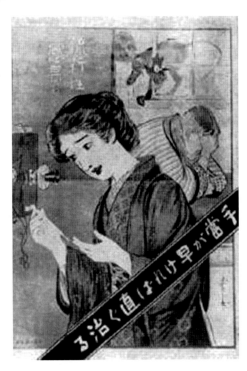

1919 Flu Victims Japanese poster. Japanese text: "If treated quickly it gets better right away."

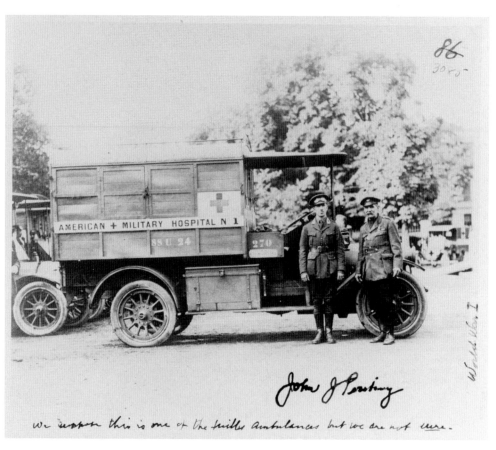

Ambulance on the Western Front. Photographed in France. This vehicle was dedicated to the memory of Richard Neville Hall. Original signed by John J. Pershing. (With permission from Naval History and Heritage Command NH-89455).

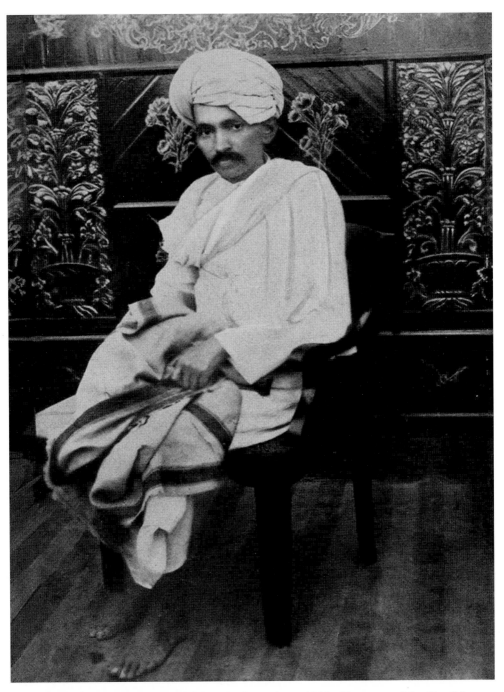

Gandhi during his support of the Kheda workers, 1918. (Courtesy of the Gandhi Book Centre, Mumbai, India).

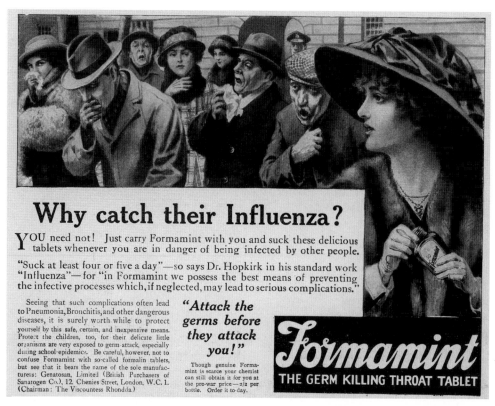

Why catch their Influenza?

YOU need not! Just carry Formamint with you and suck these delicious tablets whenever you are in danger of being infected by other people.

"Suck at least four or five a day"—so says Dr. Hopkirk in his standard work "Influenza"—for "in Formamint we possess the best means of preventing the infective processes which, if neglected, may lead to serious complications."

Seeing that such complications often lead to Pneumonia, Bronchitis, and other dangerous diseases, it is surely worth while to protect yourself by this safe, certain, and inexpensive means. Protect the children, too, for their delicate little organisms are very exposed to germ-attack, especially during school-epidemics. Be careful, however, not to confuse Formamint with so-called formalin tablets, but see that it bears the name of the sole manufacturers: Genatosan, Limited (British Purchasers of Sanatogen Co.), 12, Chenies Street, London, W.C. 1. (Chairman: The Viscountess Rhondda.)

"Attack the germs before they attack you!"

Though genuine Formamint is scarce your chemist can still obtain it for you at the pre-war price—2/2 per bottle. Order it to-day.

Formamint
THE GERM KILLING THROAT TABLET

'Why catch their influenza?'. An advert for Formamint germ killing throat tablets to ward against the spread of influenza. (*Illustrated London News* Ltd/Mary Evans)

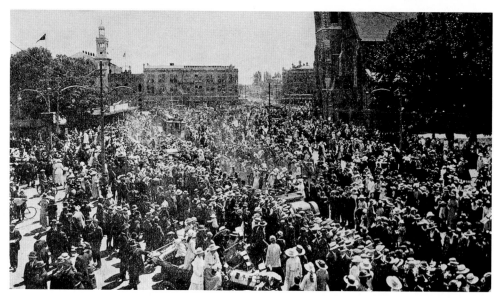

The Armistice, Cathedral Square, Christchurch NZ. With thanks to Sir George Grey Special Collections, Auckland Libraries.

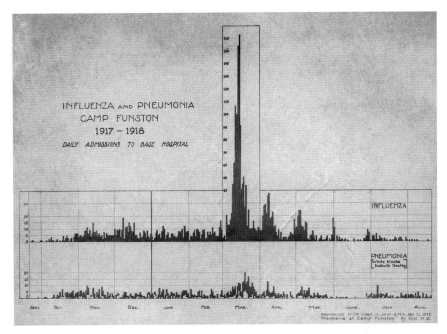

Chart of influenza and pneumonia at Camp Funston, 1917-1918. (National Museum of Health and Medicine)

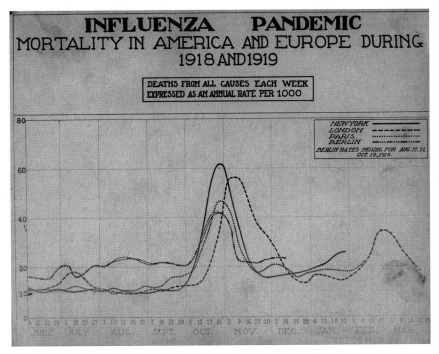

Influenza Pandemic, Mortality in America and Europe during 1918 and 1919. (National Museum of Health and Medicine)

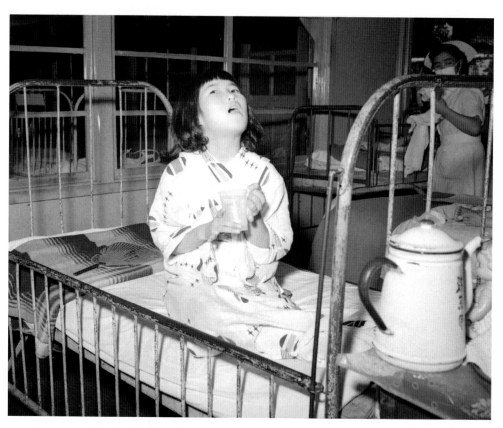

Japanese girl gargling in an influenza ward in Sagamihara Hospital, Japan, 9 August 1957. (National Museum of Health and Medicine)

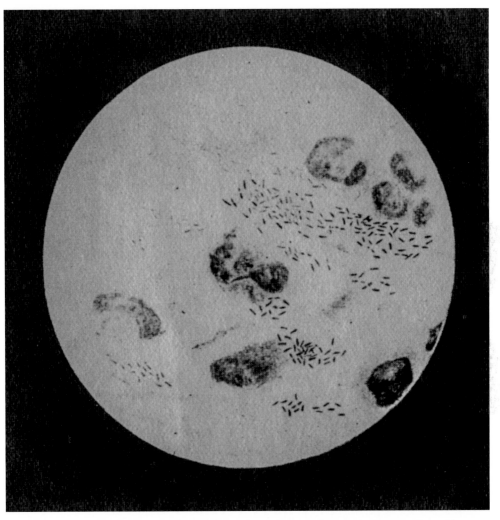

Microscope slide with bacillus influenza in sputum. (National Museum of Health and Medicine)

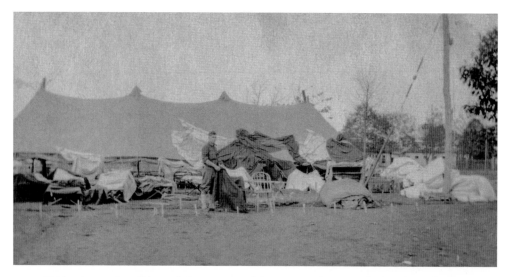

Collapsing and packing of the tents used for tent settlements during the influenza epidemic, Camp Mills, Long Island, New York, 1918-1919. (National Museum of Health and Medicine)

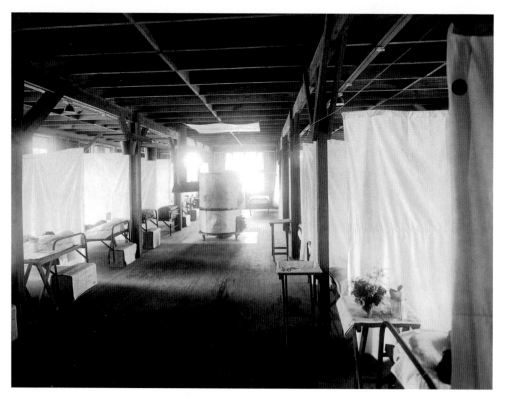

Interior hospital wards of the emergency hospital during influenza epidemic at Camp Jackson, South Carolina, September and October 1918. (National Museum of Health and Medicine)

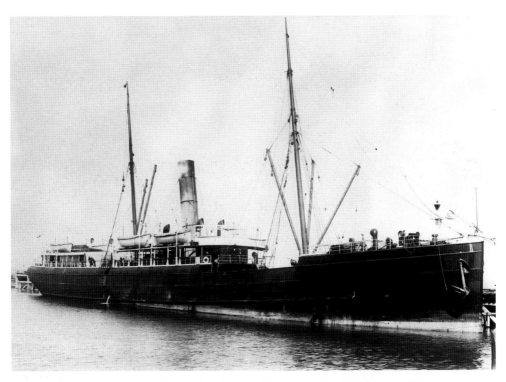

Steamship *Talune* at the Napier breakwater. (Alexander Turnbull Library, Wellington, New Zealand)

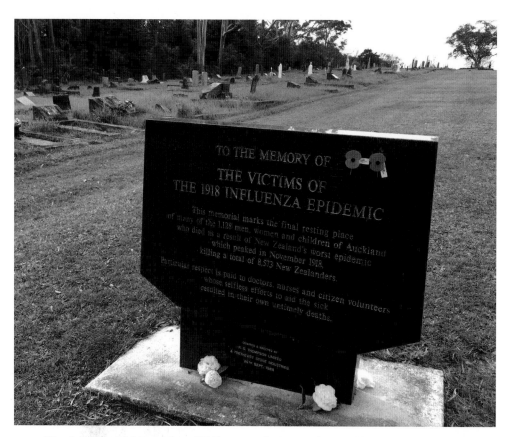

The Influenza Memorial at Waikumete Cemetary in Auckland, New Zealand.
(Jaime Breitnauer)

in some places. The Allies, still waiting for reinforcements from the US, were in a precarious position and Germany managed to gain more than 1,200 square miles of contested land in under four months, placing them dangerously close to Paris – and victory.

Around the same time that the American Expeditionary Force made landfall in France in mid-April, the first wave of Spanish flu appeared in full force among the Allies. By May, it had spread across the trenches into German lines. Given the name *Blitzkatarrh*, it put almost a million men out of action at a critical point in Germany's war. By July, it temporarily halted the previously successful German offensive (as Colonel Soltau described himself in his 1919 report to the Royal Society of Medicine) and despite having Paris in their sights, many companies were forced to pull back so that their men could recover, as in Richert's example. By the end of the month, Germany had suffered a blistering defeat at Reims and other offensives had to be cancelled. According to historian Andrew Price-Smith, German Chief of Staff, General Eric von Ludendorff later went so far as to blame Spanish flu for their loss, claiming their July offensive would have won them the war but for the fact that so many men were laid up. Historian Richard Bessel later wrote that in June and July alone, more than 500,000 men were affected, with almost 2 million affected by the flu in total between March and July 1918. Even when they returned to the Front, the German army troops were exhausted and disenchanted and a lack of supporting manpower meant the supply system was breaking down creating shortages of food, medicine and other essentials. The British took the opportunity to wage mental warfare on the stricken German troops, and thousands of propaganda leaflets were dropped by air over German lines suggesting that if their own troops could not relieve them, the British would.

Further inland, the citizens of Germany were initially oblivious to the plight of their forces. In January 1918, the government had agreed a ban on statistics relating to infectious diseases, alongside the existing wartime censorship on information around births, marriages and deaths. While there were newspaper reports as early as May 1918 about flu in Spain, little information about the situation in Germany made the press. While early outbreaks of the disease, which the German's had officially labelled influenza and declared 'minor', were reported in Nuremberg in the summer of 1918, little detail was given and much effort made to downplay the seriousness. In fact, the *Reichsgesundheitsrat* (National Council of Health) convened on 10 July to discuss this worrying outbreak and Richard Pfeiffer confirmed the disease was influenza and asserted the cause as the bacteria he had discovered some 25 years before. Despite recommendations by the Council that urgent public education was needed, information via the daily papers was still limited and the disease was not made notifiable.

The average German citizen was more worried about where their next meal might come from. The combined effects of the British naval blockade since 1914 which prevented supplies reaching the German coast, and the 'Turnip Winter' of 1916/17 when the potato harvest had failed, meant many civilians were quite literally starving. The existing shortage of food notwithstanding, a lack of manpower to assist in agriculture and the need for what little food there was to be diverted to troops had left the people of Germany to eat swedes which were usually used for animal feed. The low calorific and nutrient value left the people seriously malnourished and vulnerable to disease, with over 400,000 deaths reported as a result of famine. While the first wave of Spanish flu made only minor inroads into civilian life, the second wave which broke out in September would cut a swathe through the German populace, eventually claiming around 200,000 civilian lives.

The limited action of the national government inspired a flurry of disorganized activity among regional governments, resulting in different outcomes for different areas. In the town of Baden-Baden, South Germany, a municipal committee overseeing public healthcare made the decision to close schools in mid-October. In Heidelberg, the death toll remained relatively low, probably due to the advice that the afflicted should stay in bed. In Mannheim, the town council appealed to the Ministry of the Interior to intervene on a district office decision to close theatres and cinemas. Their major concern was for public morale as flu was, officially at least, still considered minor. The closure was subsequently lifted much to the chagrin of local doctors who complained of overcrowding in the hospitals and exhaustion among medical staff. Suggestions around 'cures' ranged from quinine to eating beetroot and inhaling onion juice. There was also great confusion about the nature of the disease, which many felt wasn't influenza despite official advice, but something related to a documented outbreak of streptococci and pneumococci. The national government maintained the official proclamation of influenza, while Pfeiffer and the Robert Koch institute in Berlin maintained their support for Pfeiffer's bacillus as the cause.

Cradling the head of his heavily pregnant wife in their Vienna home, Austrian artist Egon Schiele considered the dark irony of his situation. After years struggling to make his name, even suffering a spell in prison due to his misunderstood, often erotic art, he had recently displayed fifty works at a show in Vienna to great acclaim. After much turbulence in his love life as a younger man, he had married Edith in 1915 and she was finally pregnant after Schiele's conscription to the army had put their plans on hold. At the start of October 1918, with his career and his family on track, he might even have described himself as happy, at the very least content. But then flu struck Vienna, and his wife – whose pregnancy made her more vulnerable than she might have been – and now his hopes and dreams lay on her deathbed alongside her. Gently he sketched her, in all her vulnerability, as she lay weak and gasping for breath. It was to be his last piece of art. When Edith passed away on 28 October, ten days after falling to the affliction, Schiele already knew he had contracted flu. The same weak constitution that had saved him from active military service and allowed him to take a desk job at a POW camp had now left him wide open to infection. He died three days later, leaving behind a legacy of cutting-edge expressionism, including the unfinished painting 'The Family' – a self-portrait of himself with his wife and a child, that he had been working on during the course of 1918.

The Family is a haunting view, and not just because of the subjects' nudity and Schiele's unnerving style. It tells a story of lives unlived, of happiness unattained, which was echoed across Vienna – indeed the whole of Austria – during the second wave of the pandemic. Although the Austro-Hungarian Empire had been the first to declare war, Germany was by far the strongest force among the Central Powers. After their initial invasion of Serbia, Austria-Hungary withdrew its troops to defend its open Eastern Front against Russia and by 1916 had deferred most of the war strategy and power to Germany, who had a larger, better resourced and superior military force. As Austria-Hungary's military faded into obscurity within the wider war effort, the Empire itself began to implode. While Austria suspended government, its sister Hungary's political wheels continued to turn and its leaders were not favourable toward German military control. After the Russian Revolution, the Czech intelligentsia became restless and made their ideal of an independent socialist state well-known – an ideal that was supported by the Americans. Meanwhile Bulgaria, an ally of the Central Powers since September 1915, was forced to sign a peace treaty on 3 October 1918 after an Allied victory during the Vardar Offensive sparked a rebellion within the Bulgarian forces. On 24 October 1918, as the influenza pandemic reached its peak in Vienna, Italian forces fighting for the Allies broke through Austrian lines and Hungary resolved to break away from the dual monarchy. On 28 October, as Edith Schiele lay dying, the Czechs declared themselves an independent nation and Poland unified with the Austrian territories of Galicia and Silesia. On 29 October, a national state comprising Croats, Slovenes and Serbs was declared. The day before Schiele died, German members of the *Reichsrat* (parliament) in Vienna declared an independent state of German Austria. An armistice was signed between the now partly dissolved Austria-Hungary and the Allies on 3 November.

With all this military and political turmoil, public health went largely unattended to by the powers that be. During the course of the Great War, the weaker the grip of the Hapsburgs on power, the greater the suffering of their people. Around 35,000 Austrian civilians had already died of tuberculosis by the end of the war, according to one Austrian newspaper, with an estimated 400,000 needing treatment for the disease. Of course, tuberculosis would have left the Austrian people more vulnerable to flu and resulting complications. In the late winter and early spring of 1917, before Spanish flu burst forth on the international scene, Austria-Hungary suffered a wave of flu with a significant mortality rate possibly due to the general vulnerability of the public. Urban Austria seemed to skip the first spring wave of influenza in 1918 that weakened troops, which may have resulted in a weaker general immunity to the more serious wave that descended in the autumn. During September 1918, public transport came almost to a standstill in Vienna as so many tram drivers were struck down. Doctors found it hard to get to their patients. By October, the city had closed the schools – but it was already too late to stem the spread, and around 40,000 Austrians died. With the peak of the death toll in the two weeks before the Armistice, it has been suggested flu caused social unrest which contributed to the collapse of the Austro-Hungarian Empire, and the end of the war.

By the middle of August, the fever which had caused the German army so many problems between April and July seemed to be back in the trenches, with reports of isolated cases breaking out through the front lines. By 18 September, Spanish flu was widespread on both sides. On 26 September, Allied forces and the armies of the Central Powers stared each other down across a battle line that stretched along the entire Western Front. After their critical defeat at Reims in July, the German Army had been on the defensive, with both flu and Ludendorff's opportunist style of warfare with an apparent lack of long-term strategy considered key factors. The burden of flu on the German army was great, however, exacerbated by poor food and dwindling supply chains. So many German soldiers were affected that by June, says historian Andrew Price-Smith, medical staff were too overwhelmed to reliably record incidence. As Allied troops began their 'one-hundred-day offensive' also known as the Meuse-Argonne Offensive, Ludendorff collapsed and his staff summoned a psychiatrist, fearing a nervous break-down. Over forty-seven crucial days, the military might of Britain, America and France pushed back the Central Powers – a big turnaround from a short six months ago when Germany had been holding the better hand. Now they faced what was to be a final battle with depleted and demoralized troops and a support network that was barely functioning. Their war had become a logistical nightmare, with even the healthy debilitated by the business of flu and caring for their fellow man.

Three weeks into the offensive, German troops at the Front were once again paralyzed by flu, with up to 80 per cent of some units infected. Civilian mortality in Germany during October and November 1918 was at an all-time high, with secondary infection from tuberculosis claiming the lives of over 60,000 German women in 1918. This not only affected morale, both of troops at the Front and the people at home, but also removed a high number of previously very effective players from the German workforce. The German position seemed hopeless, and the *Oberste Heeresleitung* – high military command of the German Empire – had petitioned Kaiser Wilhelm for an armistice since the start of the offensive. On 4 October, the newly appointed Chancellor, Prince Maximillian von Baden, sent such a message to US President Woodrow Wilson and appointed a new German government with representation from all the major parties. It was Baden who fought against the changed position of the German high command a few weeks later and who convinced the Kaiser to pressure Ludendorff to resign in late October. After the Kiel naval mutiny at the start of November, it was Baden who put pressure on the Kaiser to abdicate. By this point, Baden had come down with Spanish Flu himself and was no doubt desperate for an end to the protracted – and now pointless – fighting. A reluctant politician and weakened by his malady, he prematurely announced the Kaiser's intentions on 9 November, before transferring his Chancellorship to Friederich Ebert, the leader of the Social Democratic Party.

By the time the armistice was declared on 11 November 1918, records show that more than 1.5 million German soldiers had been killed by flu, with the death toll in the army increasing by 683.18 per cent between 1914 to 1918. While some have dismissed Ludendorff's retelling of the impact of flu on the German's as a keenness to defer responsibility for their losses, the importance of the influenza pandemic at that crucial time certainly cannot be understated. The Germans failed to win the war for a variety of complex reasons, but flu played a decisive part.

Chapter 6

The Edge of War

How flu unfolded in the Americas

Standing in the doorway of his family's living room, six-year-old William Sardo sipped on a small glass of milk. He would have loved to have been sitting in the easy chair by the fire, as he did after school most days and enjoyed his milk while looking at a favourite story book – sometimes his mother would put on the phonograph and sit with him for a while. But no music was playing in the house today and the fire wasn't lit in the hearth even though there was a strong October chill. William hadn't been to school since Washington DC, where he lived, had closed them two weeks ago, at the start of October and you couldn't see the easy chair in the living room – *all you could see were the coffins.*

William lived at home with his mother, two brothers and father, who ran the local funeral home. On an average week, they might have received a few bodies which were kept out back. After being tidied up, dressed and placed in a casket, relatives could come and pay their respects. Then William's dad would hitch up the horses to the hearse carriage, carefully load in the coffin and make his way slowly through the streets, people stepping to the side out of respect, to take the deceased to their resting place. But since the first reported death in late September, the bodies had started to increase. By the time District Health Officer William Fowler closed the schools and banned public gatherings on 4 October, the Sardos had run out of space for the dead in their funeral home. Over the next two weeks, William's dad started bringing the sealed caskets inside, stacking them in the living room and eventually the hallway as well.

But why do we have to have them here? William's mother hissed to his father from the hallway as yet another casket arrived late one night. *They can't bury them fast enough. The grave diggers are sick and people are too scared to pick up the shovels themselves,* he heard William Snr explain gently. *Would you have me leave them out in the cold?*

The Sardos' space problem was about to be solved by another pressing concern – a lack of coffins. In his office in the city, District Health Officer Fowler stared at his assistant in disbelief. *No coffins? He said. What are we expected to do with the dead?* Every hospital bed in the city was taken and the morgues were jammed packed with up to 72 people dying a day. Now people were dying at home, their corpses lying in state on the dining room table while the families begged the city for help. *We can't have this*, Fowler said. *We've got coffins piled up waiting to be buried, and now we've got bodies lined up waiting for coffins!* When he heard there were 270 empty pine caskets being loaded on a train to Pittsburgh, he took immediate action, commandeering them for Washington's own use. Because the coffin manufacturers had hiked the price, he even bought them with the city purse and sold them on at an affordable fixed cost. In the meantime, he also solved his grave digger problem – by getting prisoners to dig the holes. With formal funerals banned under the law against public gatherings, it wasn't long before Washington started to see the stacks of coffins decrease.

Fascinated as he was by the spectacle, young William wasn't able to watch the day the last coffin was taken from his living room. He wasn't able to sit in his easy chair and enjoy the milk as he had craved for so many weeks. Like his siblings, he had come down with the flu and was holed up in bed. His family were so scared for him and for themselves. Only his mother came into his room to check his temperature and breathing and even then she kept her distance and wore a gauze mask. *Can I have a hug mummy?* William croaked through his fever. *When you're well sweetie, soon,* she promised, tears pooling. Thankfully, William did recover and by the start of November, the death rate in Washington DC had reduced dramatically as the second wave receded.

Recollections by survivors such as William Sardo (who died in 2007 aged ninety-five) of how the city of Washington DC was affected make grim reading but it was in fact one of the better prepared cities in the USA. The pandemic – which killed nearly 700,000 Americans between spring 1918 and January 1919 – was largely characterized in the States by official inaction rather than action. In Washington, the public authorities were fast and decisive around issues like closing public places and the Red Cross handed out gauze masks which you could be fined for not wearing; actions which no doubt minimized the death toll. In other places across the USA, authorities put a lot of reliance in the concept of 'civic duty'.

On 22 October 1918, Mayor James Rolph of San Francisco urged his city's people to wear gauze masks. *Who leaves this mask behind dies*, he told the press, a slogan he heard was printed on Italian military issue gas masks at the Front. The very next day, 15,000 masks had been collected by diligent citizens from the Red Cross, with even the local luxury Hotel St Francis instructing its linen workers to make masks for guests and employees, but it wasn't enough. The enthusiasm for Mayor Rolph's strategy was limited and 24 October saw a high of over 14,000 cases of flu, and 82 new deaths. Eventually, it was decided that mask wearing should be law for all the people of San Francisco from 29 October and those who refused would be arrested. Even with the full force of the law behind the gauze mask idea, within thirty-six hours over 160 people had been shackled for non-compliance. The majority of the city embraced the new legislation however, and by the end of the first week of November the epidemic in San Francisco was on its way out, a total of 1,600 deaths recorded. Faced with the numbers, it's easy to speculate that had the mask wearing been made law sooner, the toll could have been less.

The actions of city authorities across America seemed largely dictated by military and business priorities rather than health concerns and nowhere perhaps is this better demonstrated than in the example of New York. In NYC, flu deaths were actually below average at the start of 1918, with the weekly bulletin of the Health Department recording just eleven deaths in early January, compared to forty-nine in the same period the previous year. There was a spike in cases of flu in February,[1] although it didn't garner much attention at the time. Much of the focus of the health department by the middle of the year was on combatting venereal disease brought home by returning soldiers.

It's not that New York's authorities were unaware of the existence of Spanish flu – City Health Commissioner Royal Copeland was well versed in what was happening overseas – but when disparate flu cases began to surface in July there were other priorities to consider. New York was an enormous city of over five million people, and the gateway to America for many Europeans seeking a better life as well as a major departure and arrival point for troops. While a stripped-down, land-based quarantine had been put in place at the port in July, under heavy pressure from the military a full quarantine was shelved – it seems that the risk of flu to the public was more palatable than delaying military manoeuvres.[2] There was also commerce to consider and it's clear that authorities felt a sense of pragmatism was needed when combatting disease. Copeland's priority right from the start seemed to be to keep the city moving.

On 14 August 1918, the *Bergensfjord*, a Norwegian ship, made berth in New York's harbour and eleven of its passengers were taken to a Brooklyn hospital where they were treated but, crucially, not isolated and by early September the deadly second wave was in full swing. At the Bellevue Hospital in Manhattan, people were literally dying on stretchers in the corridors as staff tried to find space to accommodate all their patients, with children packed in three to a bed. One nurse, Dorothy Deming, compared her role to being under fire in the trenches of Europe. On 19 September, troop ship USS *Leviathan* arrived from France and was described as a 'floating hospital' by Eleanor Roosevelt, whose husband, the future US President, was so weak with flu that he had to be carried off the ship on a stretcher. Despite these desperate scenes being played out as the disease spread, Copeland did not take definitive action until the start of October.

On 4 October, the city authorities finally accepted that they were in the midst of an epidemic. Flu and pneumonia became reportable diseases. The Board of Health introduced staggered opening times for businesses in order to reduce crowding in the subways, but Copeland refused to mandate complete closure on the basis that prevalence of the disease was still low. The measure came under some criticism from the press, who noted crowding on the subways was still taking place and Copeland himself came under pressure from some larger business to renegotiate their opening times for economic reasons, which he did quite willingly. Although a public health campaign discouraged large group gatherings among other things, on 12 October, President Woodrow Wilson was allowed to lead a procession of around 25,000 people through New York City to encourage patriotism – over 2,000 people in the city died from flu that same week.

With the death toll and infection rate climbing and it becoming obvious that the hospitals were unable to cope, 150 emergency health centres were established across the city on 7 October. While some acted as clinics, most coordinated nurses to provide door-to-door care for those who had been quarantined at home. But, as the death toll peaked around October, isolation orders became almost impossible to enforce due to the sheer number of the sick and the lack of available doctors who were responsible for reporting. One of Copeland's more controversial decisions was keeping schools open, although he reasoned that in school, children were more closely monitored, had better access to medical care and could be educated on how to reduce the spread of the disease. He used a similar argument for keeping theatres open, again citing their positive use for education purposes around the outbreak and also suggested that their closure could lead to hysteria which would be counter-productive.

While Washington focused on isolation to prevent the spread, New York's technique centred around public surveillance to pick up symptoms and educating the people to change poor habits that could spread disease, such as spitting. While this course of action wasn't altruistic – the ramifications of closure and quarantine for a city of such commercial and military importance were considered just too great – New York did come through the epidemic with a lower mortality rate than many other US cities, which led Copeland at least to view their public health policies as a success. In modern analysis though, the value of the largely unreported and mostly forgotten February outbreak comes into sharper focus. A look at the geographic, age and socio-demographic distribution of the flu has led some to suggest that the earlier, milder outbreak which was considered 'seasonal' at the time, probably conveyed immunity to many who otherwise would have been exceptionally vulnerable to the more virulent strain. This would also explain the relatively low mortality rate in NYC compared to other cities of similar size.

Philadelphia was another large, East Coast city with great economic and military importance. A city of around 1.7 million, it had seen its numbers swell as transient workers taking military manufacturing jobs in local plants arrived on its doorstep. In addition, many of its medical staff headed overseas as part of the war effort – seventy-five percent of the city's surgeons were abroad. It was also home to an important naval dockyard. A strategic location for both the war and commerce, the pandemic nevertheless took residents by surprise.

America was built on private investment and war was no different. In order to be able to afford the army the US had suddenly grown from just under 200,000 professionals to 2 million volunteers, they were relying heavily on donated funds. Liberty Loans – government issue war bonds – were very fashionable, and on 28 September 1918, the city of Philadelphia held a parade to boost public morale and advertise the loans – they had a quota they needed to meet. This was the fourth Liberty Loan Drive parade and with marching bands, women's auxiliary troops, Boy Scouts and floats to showcase the military's finest equipment – including the new locally built biplane – it was a spectacle to behold, stretching for two miles. It was no surprise that 200,000 people lined the streets to see it. What perhaps is a surprise is the fact the parade was allowed to happen at all.

On 6 September, a ship had arrived in Philadelphia from the Boston Navy Yard and within hours some of the men began showing symptoms of flu. Just the day before, Dr John Hitchcock from the Massachusetts State Department of Health had issued a circular among health officials in Boston. Spanish flu had broken out at the Boston yard a week before and Hitchcock was concerned about it reaching the city's civilian population. But he had no jurisdiction over the military, who had assured him precautions were being taken to isolate cases; their priority was to keep operations moving, there was a war going on after all. Eight days after the ship delivered the disease from Boston to Philadelphia, an *Evening Bulletin* newspaper headline announced, 'Spanish Influenza Here'.

While Washington went into zealous shut down and New York played a game of chess between flu and military/commercial priorities, Philadelphia was simply in denial. Identifying the disease as 'La Grippe', a common term for generic flu, city officials claimed they were knowledgeable, well-prepared and that there was no fear of an epidemic. By 19 September, the first death had been recorded of 30-year-old naval yard worker James Keegan. Two more deaths were reported in the following days, but what remained unreported was the fact that around 1,200 people across the city had been struck down with flu, 400 at the naval yard alone. At this point, the city made influenza a reportable disease and officials must have been watching the numbers of the infected and dead slowly rising in the days leading up to the parade.

Unfortunately, City Hall at that time was a mess, with the Mayor arrested on a murder charge. There was no leadership or direction and so Dr William Krusen, director of the Department of Health and Charities, allowed the parade to go ahead. Keeping up morale and raising funds for war were, after all, important priorities at that time. Within two days of the parade Philadelphia was brought to its knees. On 1 October 635 new cases were reported in a single day. On 3 October, city authorities closed schools, theatres, bars and churches and banned indoor Liberty Loan meetings. Even then, the gravity of the epidemic didn't seem to have reached home, with the *Evening Bulletin* reporting on 4 October that there was a shortage of coffins but that it 'wasn't serious' – in reality the bodies were piling up at the morgue, with funerals indefinitely postponed. By 6 October, Dr Krusen had announced 200,000 cases of flu in Philadelphia, with just under 300 deaths in the previous twenty-four hours alone.

The first emergency hospital with 400 beds was opened on 7 October and medical students from the University of Pennsylvania commandeered to assist. One third year medical student, Isaac Star, noted that even the patients who didn't seem very ill on arrival were struggling to breathe within hours, a characteristic rattling sound heard in their chest as they gasped for air. Their skin turned purple from the lack of oxygen and most became delirious and incontinent with blood-tinged froth bubbling up from their lungs. At its peak, he said, a quarter of patients were dying from the epidemic, their bodies thrown into the back of trucks to make room in the cellar-morgue for more.

Out on the streets, over 2,000 nuns had left their convents to tend to the sick in the absence of trained nurses. Their work focused very much on the poor and African-American patients who couldn't access the main hospitals due to racial segregation. With the support of charities, a few small emergency hospitals for these groups were set up to help the sick even if they couldn't afford to pay. Many of these families could not afford to have their loved ones' remains removed and buried and at at least one emergency poor hospital location, a trench was dug outside for the bodies to lie in until they could be claimed. Eventually, the city would send round wagons to collect the corpses, asking families to leave their dead in the street as they did during the Middle Ages with plague.

By 8 October, essential services in the city could not run, with almost 500 police officers not showing up for work and 850 telephone company employees off sick, meaning they were only able to handle emergency calls. Embalmers had to be called in from the military and many families were left to dig their loved ones' graves themselves. By 13 October, more emergency hospitals had opened across the city and doctors were being called out of retirement. Eventually, 32 emergency hospitals were in operation across Philadelphia, to cope with the 150,000 cases of flu that were officially recorded between September and November 1918 – however, many more people caught flu and died without ever being seen by a doctor. There were around 15,000 deaths, 70 per cent of them people aged 10-40. By the end of October, the ban on public gatherings was lifted and schools, bars and churches re-opened, although spikes in flu continued through the winter months. Many families were left suffering extreme financial hardship having not been able to work for a month or more and there were many more orphans than the city could provide for. In spite of all this hardship, Philadelphia made its quota for the Liberty Loan Drive, raising $72,020,115 for the war effort.

Thumbing page after page of newsprint, Arthur Lapointe sighed. He had all the papers – all the ones worth reading anyway – and yet there was no mention of Canada at all. It was 7 October and the French-Canadian soldier, a once-scrawny farm boy from the small village of St Léandre in Quebec, was about to receive his stars as a lieutenant – and with those stars came the reminder of all his hard work, and of home.

It had been two years since he had tearfully left his family, shy and unsure, to sail to France to fight in this war. He had earned more than just his stars in the trenches, he had found his confidence, his strength, his bravery. Pinned down by mortar fire, bombarded by aerial attacks, steely determination had grown in him – after all, to succeed in the war was to live. But now, today, he felt that boyish sense of fear creeping back, the fear he thought he had banished for good in the mud at Ypres. His mother and father, brothers and sisters, safe at home in Canada, well, they hadn't written to him for weeks. Their letters had been all that had kept him going at some points in this terrible war, regular, thoughtful, full of stories of the little, daily successes of family life. And now, just as he had conquered his own inner mountain, they had fallen silent and he didn't know why. Then, six days ago he saw it, just a nib in *The Times*. 350 engineers were down with Spanish flu in Lac St Jean – *that was only two hundred miles from home*, he thought, the worry bearing down on him with the crushing weight of a sand bag. Since then he had scoured the papers for any mention of Spanish flu in Canada, but although he could tell you what King Alfonso of Spain's temperature was, and how many people had died in Bombay, it was like Canada did not exist.

War time censorship was an important tool and ultimately the reason for the fruitlessness of Lapointe's desperate search. The disease is thought to have entered Canada with returning troops via the ports to the east, (although the path of the Chinese Labour Corps through Canada in late 1917 and 1918 adds another possible entry point) and spread west along the rail lines, fanning out into communities as soldiers made their way home. On 8 September 1918, the first civilian outbreak was reported in Victoriaville, Quebec, but soon the whole country was swamped. Even the very remote and isolated communities which had no links with returning soldiers found themselves infected and it seems that the postal service may have been to blame there.

Canada had a famously reliable post that penetrated even to the distant north, using dog sleds when the snow was severe. An outbreak in the remote Keewatin region in December 1918 was said to have arrived in this way and the community, with little food available in the middle of winter, suffered from starvation and deaths caused by secondary pneumonia when the sick got up too soon to try and help others. As the ground was rock solid, burial was impossible in many places and survivors were forced to stack bodies inside, or even to place them on the roof, to prevent them being eaten by dogs. More vulnerable to the virus, the indigenous people who occupied these fur trading regions were much more likely to die, with entire families being wiped out across the Canadian North. Many small family units, out manning the trap lines hundreds of miles from the trading posts, would have died alone with little food and no medical help readily available to them. As the initial, virulent outbreak waned, secondary waves swept across Canada in 1919, with as many as 50,000 people dying in total.

José Paranhos, a Diretoria Geral de Saúde Pública's sanitary inspector, put down his copy of the journal *A Careta* and sighed heavily. An odd disease, the one that in Europe they called Spanish flu, had arrived in Rio de Janeiro in August, and thankfully its impact so far hadn't been that great. That didn't stop people speculating, though. Brazil had entered the war the previous year, after Germany had sunk some of their ships, but there was much public criticism around what the people had considered the government's slow response. Brazil was a proud nation and the people were also suspicious of authority. First, *A Careta* had suggested the Spanish flu was manufactured in Germany as a weapon of war and now they were claiming that it would act as a device to herald more 'official medicine' – or the government getting involved in people's private affairs. That wasn't tolerated much in Rio de Janeiro and what worried Paranhos was that he knew they would have a fight on their hands if flu were to spread.

The people of Rio viewed flu as a common disease and the influenza in Europe as something related to warfare that shouldn't affect them. This bizarre mixture of complacency over the nature of the illness and fear over the government response, would have great implications on how it was handled in the city. Although word was received that 156 people, including some Brazilian nationals on medical mission, had died from influenza on the ship *La Plata* en route to Dakar in September, the Director of Public Health, Carlos Seidl, did little to plan for the impending outbreak, partly due to the social discontent official meddling would cause and partly due to a lack of information about the epidemic because of wartime censorship. As the death toll began to grow, the city's infrastructure began to fail and both food and medicine were scarce and expensive. By 22 October, when 930 people in Rio died from flu, it was obvious the city couldn't cope, the hospitals were understaffed and ill-equipped and the city simply didn't have processes in place to deal with a mass outbreak.

It was said that there was not a single street in the city where a whole family hadn't passed away and responsibility for feeding the sick and handing out medicine was passed on to the policemen, refuse workers and those who had come to collect the many corpses piled up in the streets. Yet, among all this devastation on the ground, Seidl and the city authorities still insisted that the disease was largely benign. Seidl himself came under crushing public and press criticism for his stance. It was only on 30 September, when the disease had been raging for weeks, that authorities began to institute some measures such as emergency rescue and home assistance, but these fell well short of what was required and the medical community remained divided on what the sickness actually was. The city in chaos, incensed newspapers began running stories that not only openly criticized the city authorities, but the Wenceslau Braz government who were in power at the time. The disease became a political tool, used by opponents of the official administration to score points. With protests erupting in the streets, soon it wasn't just the people in government under criticism, but the nature of republican government itself.

Ultimately, public dissatisfaction over the way the epidemic was handled not only lost Seidl his job, but gave birth to the Sanitation Movement which, during the course of the 1920s, would completely restructure public health in Brazil and raise the importance of science-based medicine in sanitation policy. With the people of Brazil having witnessed first-hand the results of a lack of centralized funding and control over medicine, there was much more support for the public health initiatives which focused on using good science to prevent and treat disease, rather than apportioning blame for suffering onto the individual themselves – a theme that was echoed across the globe.

Although deaths from influenza raged not too many latitudes above them, much of South America did not receive a first wave of Spanish flu until the autumn of 1918, probably via the sea ports from Asia. Death rates peaked around January 1919 and in these poor countries with limited medical resources and sanitary issues, Spanish flu rumbled on through into 1920. Lima, Peru, seems to have been one of the earliest sites of outbreak, with an early spike in flu-related deaths around August 1918, although this was dwarfed by a later outbreak in January 1919. The more isolated Peruvian cities such as Ica suffered an even greater toll in 1919, when the more virulent second wave hit, most likely a result of a lack of immunity in the more vulnerable patients who had not been exposed to the mild first wave.

In Chile, the first reports of the new flu appeared in Santiago-based newspaper *El Mercurio* in October 1918 and was suspected to be typhus. With little concern over the disease, which was not thought to be airborne but rather aggravated by poor personal hygiene, public gatherings weren't curbed. Although the hospitals were already beginning to struggle with capacity issues around late October, people weren't dying the way they were in Europe and America so there seemed little need to panic. In December, after Chilean pilot Dagoberto Godoy became the first person to fly over the expansive Andes mountain range to the East in his British-issue Bristol M.1c monoplane, a huge crowd gathered in Santiago to celebrate. Within days the rate of infection in the city had sky rocketed, although the number of deaths from flu didn't peak until August 1919 and those over fifty were most affected, as in Peru.

The remoteness of South America and its lack of exposure to viruses common in Europe and Asia seems to have played a huge role in how Spanish flu played out across the sub-continent. The amount of time it took for the virus to travel to, and around, the various regions and low background immunity of inhabitants affected the number and type of victims in a way not seen in the Northern Hemisphere. The way that Spanish flu affected developing countries that had been colonized and subjugated at that time by Europeans is essential to understanding how the virus worked. It is also a lesson in appropriate humanitarian response. As we will see, the impact of flu on indigenous peoples went well beyond the terrifying death toll, resonating into the politics and equity-seeking social movements that would come to shape the world in the twentieth century.

PART 3

MOVEMENT, TRADE AND THE VICTIMS OF COLONISATION

EXPOSURE TO THE VIRUS BEYOND EUROPE

Chapter 7

Under the Desert Sun

Influenza in Africa and the Middle East

Wiping the sweat off his face, William Hill sighed deeply. He was hot, even though it was the middle of the night. He'd felt clammy since he started his shift. It was 1 October in East Rand, South Africa and Hill's job was to lower the miners of the East Rand Proprietary Mines down in the cage and then bring them back up again when needed. It wasn't an interesting job, but he had to stay on his guard – safety was paramount. The gold reefs here on the Rand were quite deep and inside this mine, which had been open for just over 20 years, there was almost no light; you could barely see a hand before your face if it wasn't for the lanterns the men carried with them. The deeper you got, the hotter it got - the rocks actually radiated heat. It was like the Devil himself lived down there and the men stole from him every day in the dark.

Most of the miners were black and travelled here from other parts of South Africa to work contracts – long, dangerous, exhausting contracts – before returning home to their mothers or their wives. It was hard work, but the money was better than you could get elsewhere, especially for the Africans. Many were young men, whose fathers and brothers worked in the mines. Many had family who had died in the mines – although safety was improving all the time. In fact, just the previous week, the cage drivers had been called together for a talk. They were, after all, directly responsible for the lives of other workers, their supervisor reminded them. There had been some strange things happening in the mines recently, men struck down suddenly with fever, shivers, incapacitated. Flu, they said it was, a minor affliction in the grand scheme of things, but it came on so suddenly, so ferociously, that since mid-September more men filled the sick bay than went down the shaft. Apparently, 14,000 men in mining operations in the Rand had come down with it and Hill had seen them setting up temporary field hospitals on his way to his shifts. While 100 white miners were afflicted, the blacks were suffering in much larger numbers. They had always been more likely to catch a cough or cold. Pneumonia was a big problem and, as they all lived together in a compound, these bugs often spread easily and quickly. *But only one person had died, and it would no doubt pass soon,* Hill told himself. Outbreaks of respiratory disease were quite familiar to the miners.

Hill wiped his face again, his eyes moving in and out of focus. *Report unusual symptoms*, the supervisor had said. *Don't operate the cage if you don't feel well ...* But Hill convinced himself he was just tired. The mines ran 24/7 and these nights shifts always hit him hardest. It was about 3.30am, only a few hours before he could head back to his bed. Just then, he got the signal that a group of men were in the cage ready to be pulled up. As he leaned forward to the controls, sweat pooled across the dimples in Hill's cheeks and chin ... He pressed the button to start the engine, it was a fair journey to the top, 100 feet, but the sweat was in his eyes now, stinging. He heard a voice ... distant ... *are you okay?* And then suddenly lights exploded before his eyes. Dizzy, head thumping, he collapsed forward into his hands. He could hear the shaft gears turning, he could hear shouting now from the men, he knew he had to stop the cage ... but he couldn't move. He couldn't reach out, he couldn't call out ... *the lights ... my head ...* Panic rose within him. Suddenly there was a terrible noise. As Hill had failed to stop the cage, it smashed into the head gear at the top of the shaft and coming away from its fixings, plummeted to the ground. Twenty men died that night in the accident, and eight more were injured. Hill was sent immediately to the medics where he was diagnosed with a sudden onset of Spanish flu and was unable to return to his duties for a month.

It was unclear how the Spanish flu made it to the gold mines of the Witwatersrand region. The first case in South Africa was in Durban, on 8 September. Some thought it had come to the North-Eastern mining region via a mail man, others said it was the migrant workers. Over a period of six weeks from the start of October, more than 60,000 men of the 190,000 working in the mines were admitted to the hospital as a result of flu and more than 1,100 died.[1] Many workers with expired contracts fled home and as news spread about the outbreak, recruiters found it harder to source men to take their place. A recruitment drive in Mozambique may have made things worse, as in mid-November when the workers arrived, they appeared to bring an even deadlier strain of the virus with them. So serious was this outbreak that the Witwatersrand Native Labour Association had halted all recruitment from Mozambique by early December.[2]

In Kimberley, a diamond mining area, the impact was even greater with more than 2,500 miners – a quarter of the working population – dying as a result of flu. The cramped working and living conditions, inadequate supply of food and lack of suitable washing facilities meant that these men were no stranger to disease, but this was like nothing they had seen before, cutting men down in packs, even the young and healthy ones who had recently arrived. It wasn't just the death toll that was exceptional, the economic impact was immense. The gold and diamond mines, severely short staffed and suffering widespread panic, recorded their profitability at a record low for 1918 – even lower than during the labour strikes of 1913.[3]

While the Rand most likely received its first flu from Durban, (a milder outbreak in July perhaps conveying some immunity), Kimberly got the more deadly form of the virus in autumn direct from Cape Town. The troopship *Jaroslav* made port in Cape Town on 13 September 1918, carrying 1,300 men from the South African Native Labour Corps home from Europe. She had previously berthed at Freetown, Sierra Leone, and since leaving, the *Jaroslav* medical officer noted 43 cases of flu on board. A month before, Freetown had been the site of the first major outbreak of Spanish flu in Africa, arriving on a British troop ship. The health authority in Cape Town decided to exercise caution, placing the sick in hospital and the 'well' passengers in quarantine for two days to monitor them for symptoms – but they all seemed to be fine. Feeling that this strain of flu was quite mild and that the people of Sierra Leone were just more susceptible to the disease, Dr F.C. Willmot from the Public Health Department consented to allow the passengers to leave. They boarded trains travelling the city and nation to go home but a day later, staff at the quarantine site began reporting flu symptoms among themselves. By 6 October, as many as 160 deaths a day were being reported in Cape Town. Willmot subsequently came under fire from the press, the government and the average man for the way he had viewed the *Jaroslav* and also the *Veronej* troopship, which docked just after the *Jaroslav* and received the same treatment. Willmot insisted that previous troop ships had also docked with mild cases of flu on board, although modern analysis of the pattern of infection does seem to suggest the *Jaroslav* and the *Veronej* were likely to be the starting points.

The rail infrastructure in South Africa, built to support primary industry, was good and Spanish flu spread quickly and effectively. As in other places, those living in remote or rural areas seemed more susceptible – they may have never been exposed to a virus before, leaving them with little or no immunity to this deadly wave. Native Africans were particularly prone to contracting the disease. In urban areas, overcrowding and poor sanitary conditions, especially among the African people, expedited the spread. Although it wasn't a notifiable disease, the newspapers reported heavily on its presence with estimates that one in two households were infected in Cape Town. However, in those early days, the epidemic seemed quite mild and was treated very light-heartedly by many people in the city. It wasn't until the first recorded death on 30 September that worry started to mount.

On 5 October, eight times the normal number of deaths in Cape Town were recorded and there were accounts of police finding people dying of flu in the streets. Pharmacies began staying open all night because of the large number of customers queueing to buy 'treatments' like aspirin and cinnamon tablets and many manufacturing businesses were forced to close due to the widespread affliction among their black labour force. Deliveries of milk and bread to wealthy white households were suspended, as were many trains and trams. Court houses had to adjourn due to officials and witnesses falling sick and the schools were not re-opened at the start of term four. The outbreak happened so suddenly and ferociously, the understaffed medical centres in the city simply could not cope.

By the second week of October, the Mayor of Cape Town had set up a committee to deal with the epidemic and over the next four weeks coordinated a relief effort that crossed the usual social boundaries. Depots were opened in fourteen wards to hand out food and medicine free of charge and volunteers made house-to-house visits, while sub-committees dealt with transport issues, burials and disinfecting the streets. Special homes were set up to care for almost 700 children whose parents were sick or had died. Six emergency hospitals were opened across the city, staffed by volunteers and equipped largely by private donations. Divisions of race, class and religion were, by and large, ignored during the outbreak. Despite the city's best efforts, though, it was estimated as many as 14,000 people died in Cape Town. Because the usual procedures for recording deaths and undertaking burials was suspended, it has also been stated this figure could be much higher, perhaps by almost another 10,000.[4] Most of those deaths happened in the two week period at the start of October and it was suggested after that the ferocity of the outbreak coupled with the limited population of Cape Town literally caused the virus to burn itself out – there simply weren't enough host bodies to keep on going at that speed.

Between 16 and 30 September 1918, five trains left Cape Town carrying over 2,700 South African Native Labour Corps troops from infected ships, as well as black workers leaving infected areas like Kimberley, to their homes[5] across the vast country. Many lived in rural towns and villages that previously had had limited exposure to the diseases of the white population. The virus swept through the areas of the Traanskei, Transvaal and into the Natal, carrying off the indigenous people in droves. In the town of Tsolo on the Eastern Cape, equidistant from the major centres of Durban and Port Elizabeth, the *Magistrate* reported on 16 October 1918 that the disease was 'rife' and that country people were being brought to a local doctor 'by wagon loads'. A week after an initiation dance near the Kei river, attended by a black worker recently arrived from Cape Town, 28 men were dead. Observers in rural areas told how whole families were wiped out, how there were corpses littering the fields where they had dropped, with no one well enough to bury them, or too afraid to undertake the task.[6] There was little in the way of an organised response to the outbreak in the countryside, due to a lack of information and resources.

By the third week in October, there were reports of men collapsing and dying on their journey home, as workers fled the infected cities and mines. White authorities in the rural regions began to panic and when the government refused a request to ban black workers from trains or put them off at the next station if they showed symptoms while travelling, some areas took the law into their own hands. The town of Lydenburg, for example, demanded the men have a medical certificate showing they were in good health before they could disembark, while Tarkastad refused to let black workers disembark at all. Other towns instituted inspections for 'sick natives', showing that while racial boundaries were temporarily suspended in Cape Town and some other larger cities, out in the countryside, divisions were heightened as white colonialists viewed the indigenous people with great suspicion, considering them to be more susceptible to disease and therefore a danger to everyone else. In return, the distrust many rural black people had for the white colonialists lead some communities to reject a lot of the advice and even medical treatment in favour of more traditional remedies. It also led some people to reject free food and other supplies, as they were concerned that they would be taxed or have to pay for it in some other way at a later date. In some places, there was open hostility to white attempts to help black communities, with the belief that the medicine and later the vaccine was some sort of poison designed to finish off black people where the virus had failed.

The death toll in South Africa was high; however, with no clear reporting system and a lot of confusion, the final number has been left to estimates only. Of a population of around six million, it is said that half a million may have died, with the burden of that figure falling heavily on the black community. Once the dust had settled however, the major impact of the outbreak initially appeared to be faith-based. With many people feeling let down by their traditional beliefs and with the death toll among white Christians seeming much lower than in other quarters, many African people found a new or renewed interest in the word of God as spread by the numerous missionaries. Many of those missionaries also volunteered to help during the outbreak, gaining an audience with communities that would otherwise have been hard to break into. In areas with an established church following, many people turned their backs on the organised European churches, disappointed by their response to the plight of the people or seeing the epidemic as a sign from God that change was needed. The result was the founding of Black Christian communities across South Africa and indeed the African continent as a whole.

Today, 85 per cent of people in South Africa identify as Christian[7] and Christianity played an important role in both establishing and ending apartheid in South Africa. The large and well-financed Dutch Reformed Church was considered the official church of the pro-apartheid National Party, and its segregation rules and use of doctrine to justify the greater rights bestowed by law on white people was instrumental in underpinning continued political discrimination. By the early 1960s though, anti-apartheid sentiment was spreading through many other denominations after the Cottesloe Consultations ecumenical conference in 1961[8] and from that rose religious support for ending apartheid laws witnessed through the 1980s and early 1990s from voices such as Anglican Archbishop Desmond Tutu, Reformed Church Reverend Allan Boesak and the Reverend Dr Beyers Naude – once a senior figure in the Dutch Reformed Church before speaking out against segregated worship. While the entangled nature of church and state was dismantled after Nelson Mandela came to power in 1994, the various Christian churches in South Africa continue to play an important social role today. Mandela himself was born in 1918, just months before the Spanish flu outbreak and his mother, Noqaphi Nosekeni was a devout Christian who raised her son as a Methodist. She founded a church in her home village of Qunu in the 1960s and although Mandela himself didn't public express religious beliefs, journalist and biographer Dennis Cruywagen has argued that he privately held Christian faith. He says Mandela's funeral followed the Methodist tradition at his own request.

Another flu legacy in South Africa was an increased interest in Western medicine from black communities, having seen after the epidemic was over that those who were cared for by European-trained doctors were more likely to survive. A separate initiative directly resulting from the epidemic was increased funding and support for orphanages and child protection to deal with the vast number of children left behind when their families fell victim to flu. These orphanages mostly concentrated on white children, with many of the black and Indian orphans being taken into domestic service, while others followed their tradition and went to live with extended family.

Spanish flu didn't just affect South Africa and a major impact across much of the African continent was famine. The flu outbreak was during the season when farmers would normally sow crops in time for the rains, but the sickness and subsequent lack of manpower meant that many crops were not sown at all and many of the ones that were, then left unattended, failed. It has been estimated that ten per cent of the population of South West Tanzania – about 100,000 people – were lost to Spanish flu[9] and it left a famine in its wake that went on to claim many more. In his paper on the topic, James Ellison notes that because of fragmented colonial structures and the tradition of oral histories in the area, the information available needs to be picked apart to get an accurate picture of what happened. The famine itself has largely been associated with the Great War and the hostilities experienced at the border of German East Africa and Nyasaland (modern day Malawi) during the war years. People talk of a hunger, a great hunger that swept across the vast plains of the British and German protectorates and illness definitely played a role in the retelling. Indeed, the very arrival of the British into the German lands in 1916 was associated with smallpox, a disease that had actually existed in Eastern Africa for generations but was exacerbated by the movement of British troops through the region.

In October and November 1918, German troops marched across the area, pursued by the British. As they went, they visited villages and requisitioned crops and livestock to feed their men. Many Africans recruited to the German military as porters deserted at this point, filtering out to a wider area than the forces themselves reached. Both the German army and the escaping African recruits carried with them viruses they were otherwise immune to, while at the same time arrivals to the region by train from ports such as Mombasa to the north also brought the flu with them. It was a convergence and by December the area was in the full grip of Spanish flu. Not only did many people die, but the temporary incapacitation of tens of thousands of people meant that the fields went unplanted. With food stores depleted by European military forces, those who survived the sickness awoke in late January to one of the most severe famines recorded in African oral histories in the entire twentieth century.

At first, talk of witchcraft was rife, with the narrative moving more toward the terms of an *ikigwaja*, or plague as time went on. Many people saw illness as a punishment for actions committed either by themselves or by ancestors and meetings were called where chiefs tried to determine blame. Funerals and sacrifices, significant public events, were banned by many chiefs to prevent the spread – a very serious step and huge breach of ancestral tradition. Ellison argues this contributed to the homogenized view of the tribesman by the British new to the area, as public gatherings were a way to display and determine difference. This contributed to their confusing treatment of locals, appointing chiefs where no right to leadership had been gained within that community and dismissing those held in high regard by their people.

The famine, known locally as 'the famine of corms', continued for two years and during this time the usual structures, rituals and routines of local society were out of kilter, with some not being acknowledged and others introduced because of the scarcity of food – but of course, the British did not understand this. British colonialists made decisions about the structure of local society and the importance of customs based on their observations during that time and those decisions went on to have consequences, lumping several tribal groups together under one unfamiliar name, reducing the importance of female healers and placing people in power who had no traditionally earned right to be there.

In Senegal, Western Africa, Spanish flu reached the French colony in early September 1918 and raged until early December, killing almost 50,000 people in the province of Kédougou, where 1.25 million people lived. Brought to Dakar by Brazilian sailors via Sierra Leone, a delay by French authorities in inspecting the ships resulted in infected passengers reaching shore before a quarantine could be established. At the military base of Ouakam, ten kilometres or just over six miles from the port, over 150 deaths were recorded before the end of November. The chief medical authority in the colony, Dr Thoulon, stated initially that the virus only preyed on the weak and was of no concern, but within weeks it had reached every settlement in Senegal.

In Kédougou, where the most complete reports were found, schools were closed and whole villages were struck at the same time with no one to care for the sick. In lower Casamance, a local man reported that every single person had been infected and around eight per cent of the population had died, the knock-on economic effect being the fact that due to a halt in agriculture and commerce the taxes would not be able to be collected. Dr Thoulon, whose initial prophecy had been proven wrong, recommended quinine, good hygiene and alcohol as treatment, with the French army giving black soldiers rum and Europeans champagne as a prescription.

Because of the fragmented colonial state systems, the tradition of oral history among indigenous populations and the way in which events are apportioned priority within those oral histories, a full picture of the experience of many of the African peoples is hard to come by. However, Spanish flu has left visible traces across African history that speak to its depth of impact. For example, in Nigeria among the Igbo people, children born between 1919 and 1921 were known as *ogbo infelunza*, the generation born after the flu, while in Rhodesia (Zimbabwe), the white colonialists stepped up segregation laws to try and keep themselves safe – it was believed that black people were more vulnerable to disease. What is clear is that Africans were harder hit than Europeans living on the continent by both disease and famine and that many remote and rural areas suffered incredible losses which far outweigh those recorded in Western countries. Around 50 million people were killed across the continent in the space of 10 months, leaving up to 12 million orphans behind.

Further north, on the Middle Eastern peninsula, British Consul General Colonel Grey surveyed the Persian city of Mashhad (now in modern day Iran). Although Persia had tried to remain neutral, it was on the doorstep of the Ottoman Empire, which had joined the Central Powers in 1915 to wage war against France, Britain and Russia. It was also a melting pot of people; a corridor along the ancient Silk Road it was a centre of trade and home to the shrine of Imam Reza, one of the twelve sacred imams of the Shi'ite Muslim tradition, making it a place of pilgrimage and worship as well. From his window in his office at the centre of the city, Grey could see quite clearly it was the home of something else too – disease. Once a jewel in Persia's crown, the crumbling medieval walls hinted at deeper issues around hygiene and cleanliness. With an open water supply vulnerable to contamination and an uneducated populace with little understanding about how disease was spread, the city was sick literally, as well as politically.

Grey had been here since the Russians' war had ended with the Brest-Litovsk treaty signing. Although on the north-eastern side of the country, away from the immediate theatre of war, this region was strategically important and the British were keen to bring it under their control. Efforts by the independent government in Tehran at centralizing issues such as public health had therefore failed, and the city had a very limited number of medical centres. The British hold on the region was strong enough to keep initiatives from Tehran at bay, but weak in other respects. The people were being bombarded, by raiding parties from the surrounding tribal mountains, by wounded Russian soldiers and by famine – there had been reports of people eating dead animals (not animals they had killed for food) they were so desperate and the price of bread had quadrupled. The city was already suffering from outbreaks of typhus and cholera and authorities were trying to halt the traditional pilgrimage to Mashhad from Pakistan when Spanish flu arrived at the end of August 1918.

A crowded, malnourished and hygiene-challenged population were the perfect target for the influenza virus and within two weeks Grey noted the whole city appeared to have succumbed. Apart from the fact there was little access to modern medicine within Mashhad's walls, the many devout pilgrims who crowded the city at this time of year tended to rely more on guidance of *Hakims* – a type of 'doctor' whose advice often included prayer, with disease often interpreted as a punishment or the result of contact with a mischievous spirit (*jinn*). It was only with the help of Ahmad Qavam, the Tehran-appointed governor of the Khorasan province where Mashhad sat, that measures to control the epidemic were able to be taken. Qavam reinstated the sanitary committee and implemented the recommendations which that committee had made the year before in 1917, during a cholera outbreak. This meant that burials of the dead were now moved outside the city walls, against centuries of religious tradition, and it was only because of Qavam's relationship with religious leaders that acceptance was gained. Qavam would eventually serve as prime minister of Persia (Iran from 1935) five times, with his first appointment in 1921. Despite his efforts, around 45,000 people came down with flu in Mashhad, with the epidemic reaching its peak in mid-September.

Mashhad probably received the flu via Russian soldiers moving south from Ashkhabad and it's likely that those soldiers were gifted the virus from the American Expeditionary Forces who had landed at the Baltic port of Archangel. As it marched steadily west toward the capital, it ravaged the rural communities, with the death toll in some areas reportedly 20 per cent of the population. Mashhad was not alone in Iran, however, in terms of disease, famine and poverty. The country, torn apart quite literally by the war and the vying of Russian, British and Ottoman armies over the years, suffered from numerous outbreaks of contagious disease, had an opium problem and repeated crop failures. Just as in Africa, military forces requisitioned what food was left for themselves, leaving a malnourished populace. Standards of education and hygiene were low and superstition high, even in the cities. Spanish flu also entered the country via British troops arriving from infected India at the Southern port of Bandar and from Baghdad in the Ottoman Empire to the west, engulfing the country on its journey to the capital.

When it hit Tehran on 24 September, it coincided with an unusually strong western wind, resulting in the condition being named *nākoši-e bād*, or the illness of the wind. By the time the Iranian authorities realized what was happening in the city, the virus had taken such a strong hold that their efforts were best used in the removal of the dead rather than treatment of the living – cartloads of bodies, mostly from the slums, were said to have been taken to the cemeteries where they were left in open piles waiting to be buried, a humiliation in Iranian culture. Many places in Persia were still trying to cope with this first wave when the second wave made land from India in the port of Bushihr and were only spared the onslaught by a few extra days due to the common use of animal drawn transports, much slower than the railways of other nations. In Kermadesh, a city swollen to twice its number of residents by Armenian and Assyrian refugees fleeing the persecution in Turkey, many people were living on the streets and the medical facilities were beyond coping. Deaths were exacerbated by a simultaneous outbreak of malaria. In Shiraz, it was reported by Sir Mark Sykes that the people gathered in the mosques to die. All cities and large towns suffered extensive paralysis of basic services, while in the rural regions travellers reported seeing bodies on the ground with no one able to bury them – villages in the Kerman district had an estimated mortality rate of up to 40 per cent. Regions with high opium consumption, such as Kerman city, had a higher rate of death. Opium wasn't just used by addicts, it was also used casually as a tonic, for relief of malaria symptoms and hunger and it was often given to patients by the *hakim*.

Spanish flu continued its journey around the country and didn't run its final course until the autumn of 1919. While there were no accurate records kept at the time, estimates have placed the death toll at as many 2.5 million people – or 21 per cent of the population making it one of the highest globally. It left the nation – indeed the whole Middle Eastern region – vulnerable, weak and fragmented as Europe began the peace accords that would see the area divided up unceremoniously and put under the protection of various European states, decisions which would morph into a century of conflict culminating in the Arab Spring of 2011.

Chapter 8

The Strange One

The epidemic in colonial India

Although it was late in the summer in India, the day was going to be punishingly hot. It was the type of day when you might have seen children playing in the grassland either side of the river Ganges, or young brides trailing their mothers to the shore with their husband's laundry to wash. On days like these, Suryakant Tripathi remembered, he had jumped into the river, allowing his whole body to become submerged, coming up for air to feel the pounding sun against his newly cooled skin. It wasn't uncommon to see groups of young men swimming here, but he knew he wouldn't find anyone today. As he walked to the river, the fields were quiet, laundry untouched, no sound of children's laughter in the air – just a smell, a putrid, lingering smell that climbed into his nostrils, embedded itself in his hair and penetrated his clothes. He wasn't sure he could ever stop smelling it again.

Tripathi, known later in life as Nirala – 'the strange one' – was a rebel, a poet, author and profound supporter of the burgeoning independence movement in India. Just 22 years old, his life had so far been sad, a fact that did not easily escape him. Born into the high Brahmin caste, he had grown up the son of a public servant in Bengal and as such had enjoyed a certain level of comfort. But his father was strict, set in his ways and often beat him. Nirala's darling mother had died when he was just a small child, never really giving him the chance to fall back on the memory of her love.

At just 16 he was married to a teenaged girl, Manohara, from rural Dalmau, and went to live with her family five days later. He remembered how, made naïve by the pleasantries of his Bengal upbringing, he imagined her village to be a wild forest, or barren desert – a completely foreign land, even though it was just a few hours away. In fact, this historical town in Uttar Pradesh was genteel and culturally rich and Nirala would lose hours sitting atop the ruins of King Dal Dev fort, watching the people down by the river and writing poetry. Although the marriage to Manohara was arranged, the love was true and even when he left to finish his studies in Calcutta, he would regularly visit the home of his in-laws and enjoy those stolen evenings with his wife, who gave him a daughter when he was 21.

As the summer of 1918 drew on, he had been planning another visit, having recently been employed as a performer in the Raja's new theatre group – a fine change from the administration work he had undertaken before. Filled with joy at being able to exercise his creative spirit, he had hoped to share his happiness with his bride. But before the trip could be arranged, he received a telegram informing him she was gravely ill.

Reading the newspapers on the way back to Dalmau, Nirala was overcome with the realization that his wife had been caught up in the deadly flu epidemic. The outbreak had begun in June, mild and distant, confined mostly to western provinces near the coast. Occasionally you would hear of someone struck down with fever or dysentery, but he hadn't paid it much heed. By July, the cases were starting to build and spread north and east. Now it was confronting him, knocking on his door. It had arrived so quickly, if only he had known time was so scarce …

Beads of sweat pooled on his forehead. He needed fresh air, a moment to catch his breath, but his walk to the banks of the Ganges was far from satisfying in that respect. There he stood on the riverbank, infected by the smell of death. The water was swollen with corpses, bodies ravaged by influenza and then placed in the Holy River with haste – with many families unable to afford the costly funeral pyre, they were left there to be taken by the water but instead were decomposing in the heat.

Turning his head away from the devastating sight, Nirala walked slowly through the village arriving at the familiar home of his in-laws. He could hear quiet sobbing inside. Taking a deep breath, he steeled himself as he walked through the door. He was too late; his wife had died – and she wasn't the only loved one the young poet lost. While walking back to his father's village, he saw his cousin's corpse being carried to the cremation site. At his house, he found his cousin's wife on her death bed, still nursing her baby girl. When the baby died, Nirala carried her tiny body to the river himself and buried her on the banks. His sister-in-law also died and his uncle, terminal with the virus turned to him and said, 'What madness brought you here?'[1]

Nirala knew this was, and always would be, the strangest time in his life. His family, he realized, had disappeared in the blink of an eye. Back at his in-laws' village he would sit and watch each day as families brought the dead to the river, a trail of corpses that surely rivalled the bodies of dead Indian soldiers from the British war.

By the time Nirala returned to Calcutta, flu was fading away but the impact lived on. Whole families had been wiped from the face of the earth, their ancestry, their stories, gone forever. The flu had touched almost everyone, in one way or another. You could catch it whatever your caste, whatever your class, and if you didn't catch it then you were probably caring for – or mourning – someone who did. For Nirala, it meant a life widowed, with great creative prowess but no compass, moving around and championing the causes of the needy. He spent the next 40-odd years trying to pull the light toward social injustice and although he admitted later that he had always had strong feelings around this, even suffering beatings from his father for his kindness towards those considered lesser men, there is no doubt the indiscriminate horrors of Spanish flu had a profound effect on his thinking.

For a long time, no great research was undertaken to determine the impact of the disease on India. As in other places around the globe, the way in which deaths were categorized by authorities at the time proved problematic for understanding their true cause. A certain amount of decoding had to be done. For example, provincial sanitary reports from 1916-20 record the number of deaths from 'fevers' at 11,134,441 for this period. As the mean figure is 4,308,356 it is safe to assume the statistics were increased by Spanish flu.[2] In the early 2000s, Indian-born health economist Siddharth Chandra, based at Michigan State University, came across some public health data for the 1918 to 1920 period in India. This later lead him to estimate the death toll to be about 18 million. This would have been about 6 per cent of the population – but not all facets of the population were affected equally, a result of the varied social and political factors across the nation. India being a British colony obliged to send troops to the European Front, coastal towns were vulnerable to the virus as they were with mustering points for returning troops. Equally, the extensive national railway system, founded in 1853 to aid trade, became an effective conduit for flu to travel inland. Across the whole country, adherence to traditions such as ayurvedic medicine and the caste system prevailed. These factors hastened the spread of disease or amplified its effects in certain quarters.

British sovereignty was a major influence in both India's exposure to the virus and its impact on the native population. Since 1858, British Crown Rule had applied to much of India and what is now Pakistan and the other areas were 'princely states', controlled by an indigenous ruler under the protection of the Crown. Many of those states were so small, they contracted their governance back to the British. When war broke out, India was required to send troops to support the Crown and over the four-year conflict, 1.4 million men of the British Indian Army fought alongside soldiers from all over the world. As well as giving up its young men to the war effort, food and medical resources were diverted to Europe and the government of the country had their eyes firmly on the state of affairs overseas, rather than on their doorstep.

When a ship arrived in Bombay in June 1918, packed to the gunwales with troops from the trenches, no one batted an eyelid. Yes, they looked sickly and tired, well what would you expect? No one suspected their malady might be deadly. As they filtered into the packed streets of the overcrowded city, they took the virus with them and, slowly at first, it began to spread. That first wave started much like any other flu virus, causing fevers and dysentery that passed in a few days with exceptions among the old and the young. As it spread through the city and moved from the West into the United Provinces (Uttar Pradesh) and the Punjab, its virulence gained pace. By 3 July, the city of Bombay recorded a daily death-rate of 230 and mass absenteeism in work places. It was the poorest India subjects who were most affected, those who lived and worked in poor and crowded conditions, while British citizens and their allies were less touched. Even in this early stage, the epidemic was driving a wedge between the citizens of India and the British Government, the latter insisting that the fever started in Bombay, blaming the lifestyle of the indigenous population for the spread of disease.

By August, the outbreak seemed to have slowed and order began to be restored in major towns. A few weeks later though, in September, came the second wave which hit the Western, Central and Northern provinces of India so hard that the British administration were forced to admit their response was inadequate. It was this second wave that proved to be most deadly. Suspicious of Western medicine, many people failed to seek treatment at all. Those who did were met with limited staff, due to medical practitioners being sent to the Front and confusion among those who remained as to the best prescription. At this point, even in Europe, no one was really sure what this virus actually was. All efforts to control the outbreak and distribute the vaccine when it became available occurred in the major cities. The remote villages, hill settlements and farming communities were largely left to cope alone due to lack of resources and infrastructure. The failure of the south-west monsoon and its effect on the crops had already put great pressure on British rule. Food shortages were widespread and there was mass immigration to cities to find work. The government response itself had inspired an uprising among some of the farmers.

Sitting in his ashram just outside Ahmedabad in Gujarat, Mohandas Gandhi was thinking about that uprising now. Not that he saw it that way. A *satyagraha* he called it, a form of active yet peaceful resistance designed to put pressure on those in power to do the right thing without causing injury, or worse. It was a theory he had developed during the twenty-one years he lived in South Africa, where he worked as a lawyer and witnessed many injustices that were the direct result of racism and imbalance of power among the people. Gandhi's friends and colleagues were broad, from many faiths and backgrounds, and that underpinned his choices in life, choices based on what was fair, rather than what the conventions of society said was right.

Having returned to India in 1914, Gandhi was acutely aware of the way power worked in his home country – with British control favouring British people and close allies – and he was determined to make a difference in a non-violent way. In February 1918, he was able to organize a *satyagraha* in his home state of Gujarat after the failed monsoon. The peasants of the Kheda district were starving in the wake of the natural disaster and yet the government was still insisting they pay land tax. With no crops, no income and little food to eat, the peasants were being crippled by this financial demand. Gandhi's plan was for them to refuse to pay the tax and to not resist the consequences. Even as all their lands and personal possessions around them were seized, their cattle sold off and the men sent to prison, the peasants didn't flinch. Not once did they resort to violence and finally, under pressure from the outpouring of sympathy by the people, the British government in India returned all their lands and suspended the tax for two years.

This success had earned Gandhi high esteem among intellectuals looking for a future leader of an independent India. He had spent much time since actively recruiting troops to join the British in the war effort, while educating the people in the art of non-violent protest. He felt that once the war was over, the help the Indian people had given Britain would support them in their claim for some level of independence. And while it was a tough road to travel, so far, he felt progress was being made. He nodded to himself now, but his aching neck made him sit back in his bed. For the last few days he had felt overwhelmed by a sickness more severe than anything he had experienced in his 48 years. Unable to continue with his recruitment, he had resolved to rest and to starve himself to keep the bug at bay. Just then his wife, Kasturba, walked in and Gandhi could smell the appetizing aroma of the sweet porridge she loved to make. It was true, she was an excellent cook, and this was one of his favourites. Feeling weakness in his resolve, he sat up and accepted the porridge gratefully and relaxed back into his cot, dozing, his stomach full. An hour later though he awoke abruptly and knew immediately the porridge had been a mistake. He was overcome by an acute attack of dysentery that led to several weeks in bed unable to eat, drink, read or even think. Later, in his memoirs, Gandhi would record that all interest in living had ceased.

It was around this time that the government, under heavy criticism from the Indian press, appealed for help. The perception of the Indian people was that British officials had run for the hills and left the people to cope alone. The dichotomy of suffering between those at the top and those living in the dust emboldened the already vocal supporters of an independent India, with the journal *Young India* stating that although the government claimed to be the *maa baap* (mother and father) of the people, they had chosen 'to throw them on the hands of providence', while letter writers to the *Times of India* demanded to know what highly paid government officials were actually doing to help. The failure of early crops and the British insistence on exporting grain to Europe to feed the troops resulted in widespread famine, which no doubt contributed to the ravages of the virus. Although the government halted the exports in October, the populace was already vastly weakened and the rural areas struggled – and in many cases failed – to sow the next seasons crops. An exceptionally hot and dry year, there was also a mass shortage of water. In the city of Ahmedabad, where Gandhi and other prominent members of the independence movement lay paralyzed by feverish malaise, 3,527 deaths occurred during the months of September and October alone. The January 1919 report of the city health officer noted a higher mortality rate among the 'low castes' who were poor, less educated and traditionally were less likely to be helped or seek help. The independence movement, however, cut across these social divisions and, responding to the government's plea, no doubt brought relief to many under-privileged people whose suffering was greatly lessened as a result. While Gandhi languished well into November, unable to shake the sickness off, his followers answered the government's call and filled the gaps where the authorities had been unwilling or unable.

The Gujarat Sabha organization had helped Gandhi instigate the *satyagraha* in Kheda, and now they set up a group to help coordinate local relief in Ahmedabad. Supported by a local businessman, Seth Jamnabahi

Baghubhai, they were able to open a hospital with 125 beds. School teachers volunteered to make house to house visits to reach those unable to travel. In addition, they set up 24 dispensaries around the city and funded the Salvation Army to travel to villages on the outskirts of the city and some neighbouring districts. While the people of Ahmedabad seemed to suffer at the hands of the impotent regional authority, there was much wider cooperation between officials, Indian volunteers and organizations like the St John's Ambulance in other cities. In Bombay, the Hindu Medical Association took the lead among the NGOs with volunteers making house visits under the guidance of doctors and temporary hospitals being set up in Jain hostels to serve mostly the poor mill workers. The Social Service League set up the Influenza Relief Committee and used donated funds to open twenty centres across the city to distribute milk, clothing and medical supplies. Twenty-five organizations provided 200 volunteers while many other businesses, community groups and individuals offered space to organize and donations of needed items and money. In Karachi, donated funds were used to establish twelve mobile dispensaries along with free medical treatment and volunteers disseminating information about recovery and preventative measures. In Hyderabad, the Citizen's Influenza Committee joined forces with the Salvation Army to bring local relief.

In Surat, a city almost 300km south of Ahmedabad, the ashrams of brothers Kalyanji and Kunvarji Mehta and of Dayalji Desai – all three supporters of an independent India – set up a free dispensary, delivered flu relief to the houses of those unable to come to the ashrams and set about removing corpses for cremation. The fact that the Mehta brothers and Desai were working together at all was a triumph of Gandhi's call for reforms. Desai was a Brahmin and under the social norms still prevalent in India at that time, would not usually have associated with the lower caste Mehtas. But both the call for independence and the flu pandemic cut through the noise of centuries of tradition to take a more pragmatic approach that was felt far and wide. When their students took ayurvedic medicine to the remote villages, they were not initially welcomed. The students belonged to castes that had traditionally been oppressive of these 'tribes' and at first they refused their medicine, but the kindness and perseverance of the students resulted in a change of heart. The willingness of groups with links to the independence movement to reach out and help where the British government had not strengthened national ties and, for many, set a resolve in that direction. This was the power of the people of India after all.

While the people on the ground, Muslim and Hindu, were uniting, the weakened British government were pushing back. Although the war may have ended in Europe on 9 November 1918, in India, the viceroy's legislative council recommended extending wartime legal restrictions on the populace. This would, among other things, allow authorities to arrest and incarcerate those suspected of sedition without trial. It served not only to remove some basic rights from the average Indian, but also to suppress political expression at a time when the calls for independence were growing strong. While the people had perhaps been willing to tolerate the suspension of their civil liberties during wartime, the continuation of this intrusion on their rights through peacetime was not well received. When these recommendations, named the Rowlatt Acts after Justice Sydney Rowlatt, who penned the original report, became law in February 1919, Gandhi called for *satyagraha*.

On 6 April 1919, a general strike was declared across India aiming to show the people's discontent with the Acts. The result was many arrests of prominent Indian leaders which sparked protests over the next few days. One of the measures taken to restore order was a ban on public gatherings. On 13 April 1919, a group of around 10,000 people came together in the city of Amritsar, in an open space called Jallianwalla Bagh with high walls and only one exit. It was partly a celebration of the spring festival and partly peaceful defiance of the authorities. Many families who had travelled from surrounding villages did not even know of the ban. The British response was brutal, by anyone's standards, with troops commanded by Brigadier General Reginald Dyer opening fire on the unarmed gathering without warning. The result was a bloodbath and although official reports placed the death toll at just under 400, other estimates put it much higher.

Gandhi had only just recovered his strength from his bout of Spanish flu when he received the news. To say he felt betrayed was perhaps an understatement. After all, he had supported the British Raj and recruited troops to fight under the Union flag. His hopes that this might soften the sovereign view of India, he realized, had surely been misplaced. He felt his resolve harden and ramped up his *satyagraha* campaign, requesting non-violent non-co-operation with the British from all the Indian peoples. Six months before, when he had merely hoped for self-governance, support had been localized and grew slowly. Now though, in the wake of this atrocity, his proclamation that the goal should be complete independence from British rule was well received. Having united to fend off flu and been well-cared for by supporters of an independent India, the people flocked – spiritually speaking – to Gandhi's side. For the first time, he had strong, grass roots support, as the people of the country embraced the idea that a government that could let millions perish of influenza would never be sympathetic to the needs of the Indian nation. By 1921, the independence struggle was in full force with Gandhi at the helm and although it took twenty-six years, ultimately, he achieved his goal.

It's not hard to see Spanish flu as a decisive moment in Indian national history, where Gandhi emerged as a true man of the people and the British were exposed for their lack of understanding of the citizens they were meant to protect. It led to raised tensions, which led to hard politics and brutality and, finally, the alienation of the people from British rule.

Chapter 9

Closed For Business

Influenza in the South Pacific

On the morning of 8 November 1918, eighteen-year-old Ida Reilly[1] was making her way to work down Queen Street, Auckland. It was a clear spring day in the southern hemisphere and the blue sky was clearly visible between the three and four storey stone buildings lining the long, wide business avenue in the city centre. It led right down to Queens Wharf where the ships docked. As a child, she had enjoyed watching a steamer arrive from some far-flung land; it was quite the occasion and even now she would sometimes drift down in her lunch break and watch the military ships making port, wondering where they had come from and how long it had taken. It was a reassuring reminder of just how far New Zealand was away from that horrid war.

Recently though, she hadn't had much time to visit the wharf, or pay any attention at all to what was happening on Queen Street. She had been working double shifts at the telephone exchange, starting at 7am and finishing at 10pm, with just a two-hour break in the middle of the day. *So many people had come down with this flu, see, Auckland Telephone Exchange are terribly short staffed*, she had told a friend. *And at a time when people are relying on the telephones more than ever!* Since the middle of October, people had been dropping like bowling pins around the city from a mystery illness that seemed to have come from nowhere. There had been some terrible reports. Mothers lying delirious next to their dying children, whole families dead at home, undiscovered for days. At work, many of the staff had been hospitalized and Ida dreaded the news that some well-loved colleague may have passed. Even though people had been told not to use the phones unless it was an emergency, for a doctor or a priest, they would get the occasional call, a desperate and isolated soul struck down with the flu who just needed to hear a friendly voice.

Tragic though it was, being needed made young Ida feel terribly important. She even got driven home in a car after her last shift finished at night! Sometimes businesses who relied on the telephone exchange to operate would send a basket of fruit to say thank you, much appreciated by all the girls. And then there was Cookes, the local milk bar. If they needed to eat, they could put a sneaky call in – the supervisors would turn a blind eye – make an order then rush down there and find their order waiting for them.

Before the outbreak, Ida found her stroll to work down Queen Street quite pleasant. There was always an early morning bustle she enjoyed. But since all this happened, well, the street was quite quiet, compared to normal. The whole of Auckland was. The few people you did see walked slowly and sadly, heads lowered in despair. The only things moving at speed were the ambulances and then of course there were the hearses. More hearses than she had seen in a lifetime, taking the dead on their final journey. Yesterday, the government had closed the schools, so you couldn't even hear the sound of children playing at lunchtime. It was so lonely and Ida didn't stroll to work anymore, but would hurry, not just because she was needed but because she needed to get off the streets, into the cover of the exchange where warm friendly faces were abundant.

This morning, though, she stopped suddenly, her eye caught by something exciting but strange. Outside the offices of the *New Zealand Herald* newspaper was a sign declaring the war was over. Apparently, a cable late the previous night from America had shared the good news that Germany had surrendered – although the government had refused to confirm it. As she stood there, reading, Ida realized people were standing around her, a crowd was growing. She turned to see more people gathered around the sign than she had seen on the street in weeks. A murmur rippled through the crowd, *the war is over, the war is over* … then out of nowhere someone let out a cheer. Suddenly church bells were pealing and the streets filled with excited Aucklanders, some who had not left the house for many, many, days, some of whom had got off their sick bed and were coughing and spluttering all over the crowd as they joined in the celebration. People were laughing, crying, strangers were hugging each other. It was so unusual, but an incredible sight to behold.

Ida smiled, her heart full of joy. *Thank goodness, this madness has come to an end*, she thought. She did not allow herself to get carried into the crowd though. Excited as she was, she still had a job to do and she hurried off down the street to the exchange. The celebrations continued without her nonetheless. For hours, people walked Queen Street, shaking hands, embracing. Impromptu bands played on the corner and Union flags sold out completely. As news spread into the suburbs, people walked into the city to join in the fun.

Sitting in his temporary office in Auckland, Acting Chief Health Officer Dr Joseph Frengley was horrified by what he saw. Apart from the fact that he knew, by direct line to government, that the armistice news was false, the way people were coming together would only aggravate the spread of this terrible disease which they were yet to get under control. He had done so much work, so much good work since his arrival on 3 November, even persuading the Minister of Health to come up from Wellington to inspect the situation, which had resulted in the declaration of influenza as a notifiable disease. He had issued notice of the temporary closure of public gathering spaces, like public halls and shooting galleries, set up inhalation spray points around the city where people could pass through atomized zinc sulphate spray and brought in military doctors to replace stricken GPs in areas with no medical care. It was he who had closed the schools just the day before. He had thought they were making progress – until this.

Thankfully, he had a bullet in his gun. Section 18 of the Public Health Act allowed him to declare that proprietors of shops, hotels and similar establishments close at 4.30pm, and he dispatched the police to break up the crowd. A few days later, on 12 November, because of the time difference, when the real armistice was declared, Frengley banned any public celebration. While other cities in New Zealand enjoyed carnivals and parades, the streets of *Tāmaki-makau-rau* (the Maori name for Auckland) were silent, except for undertakers and funeral processions. There were 83 deaths on that day, the highest during the city's outbreak, with just over 1,000 people dying in total – seven per cent of Auckland's population. The mortuary overflowing, Victoria Park in the city centre had to be used as a temporary, outdoor morgue.

Frengley's concern around the celebration's ability to spread the mystery flu probably did Auckland a huge favour. While two death trains a day took the bodies of Spanish flu victims out to Waikumete Cemetery in West Auckland between 13 and 20 November, by the end of the month there were less than ten deaths in the city per day. This was not the case in other New Zealand localities where the disease spread rapidly after Armistice Day. While Christchurch, a large city on the South Island, had suffered its main – and comparatively mild – outbreak earlier than Auckland in October, many in the nearby rural settlement of Temuka in South Canterbury came down with flu after Show Week, 6 to 9 November. Many would have travelled to Christchurch for the event. On 12 November, the community came together to celebrate the armistice. Although the recent death of two sisters from flu was fresh in everyone's mind, continued war time newspaper censorship resulted in many communities not understanding the extent of the crisis in the major towns. They knew more about what was happening in Europe than in their own country. Deaths from flu complications weren't unusual in the early twentieth century, especially in rural areas and although the Rickus sisters who lived in the nearby Maori settlement had not been in the usual demographic – they were 29 and 33 years old – the wider community hadn't paid the news much heed. The Armistice was far more important and the day rolled on with speeches, processions and the entire town rejoicing in the streets.

On 14 November, well respected local sheep breeder Donald Grant died. He had been at the show in Christchurch but came home early to Temuka after being struck down by flu.[2] The same day, the borough council held a special meeting to organize a response to the local epidemic. The Presbyterian Sunday School Hall was commandeered as an emergency hospital and the Red Cross volunteers became the nursing staff. Forty-eight hours later there were over twenty patients inside. Printed advice was distributed door-to-door and a local was sent to collect a Health Department nurse from Arundel, 30 kilometres or 20 miles away. Nurse McMahon was charged with attending to Maori patients at the Arowhenua settlement and a separate hospital was set up at the Anglican Parish Hall by Sunday morning with the Salvation Army Hall being used for convalescence. A week after the Armistice celebrations, the town was silent and closed under the shadow of influenza. By 9 December, though, there were only two cases left in the hospital and no new admittances for days. Seventeen of the 1,633 residents of Temuka district had died – nine of them from the small Maori settlement.

The experience of Temuka was fairly typical of that in New Zealand as a whole, with a few notable exceptions. The settlement of Te Araroa employed roadblocks and locals with shotguns to prevent people entering until the outbreak was over, while boarders at Nelson Boys' college set up camp in the bush at Maitai Valley until they got the all clear. The Armistice celebrations seem to have aggravated the extent of the outbreak in many regions. University of Canterbury Emeritus Professor of History Geoffrey Rice notes that the willingness of local authorities to eschew official Health Department warnings and continue with the Armistice celebrations demonstrates the very casual attitude that people had towards flu at the time. It was not seen as a serious disease.

While the authorities were well informed, the lack of information available to the public was another aggravating factor. Wartime censorship meant that early reports of flu were suppressed and citizens of New Zealand were left without fair warning about what they were dealing with. This also made tracing the origin of the epidemic difficult. Many blamed the arrival of the RMS *Niagara* in mid-October. Having sailed from Vancouver carrying the New Zealand Prime Minister William Massey in September and arriving in Auckland with several severe cases of influenza on board, it seemed obvious to many it had brought a new disease with it. But as Rice notes, there was no influenza outbreak in Vancouver when the ship left, nor at any of the ports where it berthed along the way. In addition, several military vessels made port in Auckland both before and after the *Niagara*. An official Health Department report, authored by Dr Robert Makgill in 1919, notes the short incubation time for influenza of just 48 hours compared to the fact that the main outbreak happened in Auckland 14 days after the *Niagara* docked and three to four weeks later in other parts of the country. In addition, there had been deaths from flu as early as 6 October, well before the ship arrived. He felt the timeline didn't make sense, the *Niagara* couldn't be the delivery boy and the virus present in the country must have already been mutating into a more aggressive form. Today, it seems more likely it found another route in on a military ship.

During the severe second wave of influenza that swept New Zealand in October, November and early December 1918, Emeritus Professor of History Geoffrey Rice reports that Maori were seven times more likely to die than Europeans, a curiosity also reflected in other non-European populations overseas. The Maori peoples arrived in New Zealand – which they call *Aotearoa*, or Land of the Long White Cloud – around 1300CE. Legend has it they sailed on a giant ocean-going *waka* (canoe) from *Hawaiki*, their mythical homeland to where spirits also return upon death. Genetics place their origin in Polynesia. The most important fact to consider is that the Maori lived in isolation for centuries, a small population on a distant, untouched land. It wasn't until Europeans began arriving in the seventeenth century that they became exposed to other cultures, languages, foods and, crucially, diseases.

Measles, whooping cough and the inter-tribal wars of the early nineteenth century had already more than halved the pre-European Maori population. It was thought to be recovering until the flu pandemic hit New Zealand's shores. But the Maori people, who by and large continued to live rurally and away from European settlements, had a low exposure to common colds and mild flu viruses, resulting in a lower general immunity to new virus strains. At that time, Maori people also lived in their traditional style, sleeping in large groups in close quarters where a virus could easily spread. Some Maori settlements were greatly impoverished due to having their land taken; their poor diet, low quality housing and lack of access to medical professionals or supplies also increased their vulnerability. Rice says that European ideas about disease were slow to catch on and many attributed the disease to supernatural causes which led to a kind of 'fatalism' described by many relief workers, who told how many Maori patients 'just turned their faces to the wall and died'.

The plight of Maori influenza victims weighed heavily on the New Zealand administration, as did that of the working class *Pākehā* (European) victims – many of whom were living in squalid conditions in what relief workers termed urban slums. The pandemic of 1918 formed a platform for a swathe of reforms in New Zealand, the crowning jewel of which was the Health Act 1920 which formed the foundations of the public health system New Zealanders enjoy today. Elsewhere in the South Pacific, other indigenous populations suffered a similar fate but in some cases with much less sympathy from their imperial protectors.

When the SS *Talune* made port in Apia, Western Samoa, on 7 November 1918, the New Zealand protectorate's administrator, Colonel Robert Logan, made no attempt to impose a quarantine. He had governed the Western Islands since they were seized from Germany at the start of the war and had seemed sympathetic and well-versed in local custom, restoring many of the civil liberties the Germans had taken away. Yet, even though he was aware of the outbreak of Spanish flu in Auckland, *Talune's* point of origin, that information was not passed on to the port's health officer and passengers were allowed to disembark with impunity.

The outbreak was swift and vicious. Samoans had limited exposure and therefore no real immunity to flu and their tradition of the family gathering around the bed of the dying and the dead expedited the spread. Within a week, flu had reached every part of Western Samoa – and Robert Logan seemed not to care. He had made no attempt to quell the spread and refused medical help from the neighbouring American-controlled Eastern Islands of Samoa, whose own quarantine had been effective. When the New Zealand medical officer and his wife tried to set up aid stations, he insisted they be shut down.[3] Entire families died with such speed that their bodies lay around for days, even weeks, until the New Zealand army either threw them in mass graves or torched their houses on Logan's instruction – no concessions to traditional practices or beliefs were made. Many of the dead were the *matai*, the elders who led their communities, and this was to be a key factor in Samoa's future. Whether Logan was overwhelmed by the enormity of the situation, or just didn't care is still up for debate, but his failure to take the threat seriously, or introduce any official response, no doubt exacerbated a terrible tragedy. In the space of a few months Western Samoa lost around 8,000 people – 22 per cent of their population – and although Logan was replaced as administrator, survivors became hardened to New Zealand rule.

During German occupation, citizens had used the principles of *Mau*, or non-violent protest, to highlight their discontent. Now, as deceased elders were replaced by younger *matai* who were more disgruntled and more familiar with European ways, the Mau movement saw new life. Building their offices by the mass graves of those killed by influenza, the movement grew in strength throughout the 1920s, with the majority of Samoans participating in acts of civil disobedience which included refusal to harvest crops like coconuts, refusal to use official registers for births and deaths, refusal to pay taxes and boycotting of imported goods. When a large military force was sent to try to put an end to the resistance, so many people offered themselves freely for arrest the New Zealand authorities were unable to cope. On 28 December 1929, ten years after the Spanish flu epidemic ravaged the islands, New Zealand military police fired on a largely peaceful Mau demonstration, killing eleven people and wounding fifty more. A truce between the Mau leaders and the military police was called in March 1930 and when a Labour government was elected in New Zealand six years later, efforts to contain the Mau were largely relaxed. The people of New Zealand expressed unhappiness at the way their government had dealt with the Samoan protectorate and in 1962, independence was finally gained.

Political unrest as a result of Spanish flu was also a theme in Australia, which was still trying to find its feet as a federation. While New Zealand may have appeared closed for business during the pandemic, its cousin over 'the ditch' (the Tasman sea), actually *was* closed with quarantine imposed on every port. Having watched this terrifying disease creep closer and closer to their shores since mid-1918, Australian officials took early action, introducing quarantine measures at the start of October 1918.

Scanning cabled reports from New Zealand during November and early December, Director General of the Commonwealth Quarantine Service, Dr John Cumpston felt pleased with a decision he knew some quarters had found extreme. New Zealand, after all, had just as much warning as they did, but had chosen to rest on its laurels a little more than Cumpston had been comfortable with. A mild autumn outbreak across Australia earlier in the year had been hard enough to deal with. He knew that this new, more vicious influenza reaching Australia's shores as summer in the southern hemisphere began would be a disaster.

Australia was a very young nation, having only formed its federation of colonies in 1901, under British dominion. In addition, this outsized continental land-mass had a tiny population, with remarkably long distances to travel between most urban populaces. Therefore, each state took responsibility for its day to day governance, while the Commonwealth looked after the federal structure that knitted the states together. While this made sense in many ways, it did mean there was little national agreement on certain things, one of those being public health. Unlike New Zealand, which was one of the first countries in the world to have a public health department in centralized government, each state took responsibility for its own. Cumpston, and other Federal officials had seen the need early on for a more unified approach to Spanish flu and at a meeting in November 1918, all the states had committed to thirteen resolutions designed to ensure they acted cohesively, quarantine being one of these.

For a short time, it seemed the quarantine had worked – by Christmas, the Aussies were still sitting pretty. Then, in early January 1919, there was a suspected case in Melbourne, Victoria. It was so mild, though, surely nothing to worry about? It hadn't even been officially confirmed as Spanish flu by Victorian medics yet and even when several more suspected cases cropped up over the next week or so, Victoria was not pushed for a declaration of outbreak by Cumpston. Victorian authorities themselves held back on notifying colleagues in other regions and strategies around first response inland were delayed.[4]

On Saturday, 25 January, residents of otherwise unaffected Sydney, New South Wales, woke up to read news reports of a suspected case in one of the suburbs – a soldier who had arrived in the city from Melbourne. By 27 January, there were several positively identified cases and NSW became the first state to declare an outbreak, with Victoria finally following suit the next day. Melbourne's actions angered some officials, as it went against the agreement at the influenza planning conference in November. They also felt let down by Federal government, who were meant to take responsibility for communicating an outbreak. Now, the various states' confidence in the Federal power of the Commonwealth was severely shaken, and they abandoned the November agreement, shutting state borders and dealing with their own outbreaks in the way they saw most fit.

The resulting mis-match in policy across the country caused some very curious outcomes, not least in the small town of Tenterfield, New South Wales. A border town with rural farming community of about 1,000 people, the mail train from Sydney to Brisbane, Queensland passed through here. On 25 January, just hours before Sydney declared its outbreak, the mail train left for Brisbane also carrying passengers returning home after the Christmas and New Year celebrations. When Queensland heard news of the outbreak, it closed its borders – even to its own residents, something that went against the November agreement. As a result, 350 Queenslanders were unceremoniously dumped at Tenterfield after Queensland refused to accept its residents home. It was hard for this tiny settlement to find food and shelter for the crowd and the Mayor of the town sent a telegram to the NSW authorities asking them to make sure this incident wasn't repeated – but it was. More passengers left Sydney on the Brisbane mail train, and were let off at Tenterfield, and eventually 800 refugees flooded a town that simply didn't have the resources to cope or any real support. Newspaper reports described men living in a horse carriage and people destitute on the streets, but no solution could be found due to tension between the states and the Commonwealth. Eventually Cumpston and the Commonwealth had to rescind control of quarantine on land, focusing on the pre-November agreement jurisdiction of shipping. As a result, Queensland and NSW were able to agree to the establishment of two quarantine camps where residents spent seven days before being allowed home – even though they had already been in Tenterfield for several weeks.

In Western Australia, the impounding of a trans-continental train fired up anti-commonwealth sentiment in the goldmines, while in Tasmania one member of parliament suggested they should petition the king to suspend the constitution. The breakdown of high-level communication coupled with the large number of people trying to move around the country in the post-holiday period certainly heightened political tensions and put strain on the relationship between states and the governing Commonwealth.

Some argue that Australia's strict quarantine was a success, with it keeping the deadly second wave out completely and that the January outbreak was a mid-weight third-wave let in when they thought they were safe. Cumpston himself was sure Australia's epidemic in January was a mutation of the first wave, not a visitor from beyond their shores – but he was perhaps the only one who ever held that view. Spanish flu eventually killed 12,000 Australians against a population of just over 5 million – less than one per cent, compared to one to two per cent of the population of

Europe, and as many as six per cent of the global population. While each death is a tragedy in its own right, the larger statistical picture is of a nation that stayed the hand of the disease long enough to allow its virulence to weaken. While the response in the early weeks of January 1919 may have contributed to the spread, the resulting policy change lead to a robust, unified, federal approach to public health in Australia that continues today, with Cumpston himself appointed the first ever director general of health in March 1921.

Chapter 10

Closing the Loop

Outbreak and immunity in South East Asia

By the time people in China started dying of flu in 1918, Dr Wu Lien-teh had recovered from his angina attack and was president of the fairly recently formed National Medical Association. After the mysterious 'winter sickness' of 1917, many Europeans were quick to point the finger east (and many still do) when it came to finding the birthplace of Spanish flu. There was still dubious uncertainty hanging over Dr Wu's proclamations of a 1917 pneumonic plague in Shansi. In Shandong, in north-eastern China, the CLC men at the Tsingtao depot were reporting mild flu symptoms in January 1918. As late as March 1918 in Nanking near the port city of Shanghai, Western doctors reported a slow but steady parade of deaths, but none of the dead showed any signs of plague.[1]

However, when the 'new' virus set in later in the year, Dr Wu's studies of its characteristics showed it to be the same as the one raging across Europe; British reports from missionaries stationed in China at the time agreed. China suspected it had been introduced to the country via foreign troopships and men returning from the Chinese Labour Corps at the Front. Early summer outbreaks appeared on the eastern seaboard of the country, in Canton (now Guangdong), Shanghai and the British port of Hong Kong. Hopei (now Hebei), north of Beijing and close to the border with Russia were also hit. But deaths were minimal. Between June and September 1918, there were just under 300 recorded deaths from flu in the Shanghai International Settlement among a population of just over 800,000.[2] The second wave of the pandemic seems to have taken a greater toll, although it was still concentrated in the eastern and southern provinces. But the more rural the location, or the further away from the foreign controlled ports, like Hong Kong in the south and Manchuria in the north-east, the more severe the influenza seems to have been and the more likely it was people would die.

The *Tai Gong Boa* newspaper in Gejiu city, inland in the south of China, reported the outbreak reaching them in September, with at least half the city down with flu and thousands of patients dying. It was described as the worst epidemic for decades at the same time as a British physician in Shanghai, Dr Stanley, reported a high rate of infection but a limited number of deaths in the province. Scattered reports from villages outside of Gejiu painted an even more dire picture – in one village it was said that funerals were occurring daily, in another village more than half the residents were afflicted. China at that time was a mix of very traditional regions that had little to do with the outside world and provinces that had embraced industrialization and foreign trade. Large areas on the eastern coast had been annexed by foreign powers and it was in those areas, where exposure to previous viruses' was probably high, that it was said few people died – and it was noted few foreigners came down with the illness at all.

At the end of October in Hopei, local authorities announced that flu was present in the district, but that it could be kept under control with simple measures. They suggested daily cleaning of the house and spraying with limewater and to drink soup made from powdered mung bean and rock sugar several times each day. Around 5,000 doses of a herbal formula were distributed to those already afflicted and at the end of the outbreak they reported a recovery rate of almost 97 per cent – more than twice as many patients recovered in Hopei than in San Francisco.

In December 1918, a Western doctor who had been sent by the British to ascertain what was happening inland, reported from the far north-western province of Sinkiang (Xinjiang) that Spanish flu was present. He describes how it came over the border with workers returning from the Russian poppy fields and spread quickly, with at least one settlement being wiped out completely. In the city of Urumchi (Urumqi), it was reported that all shops and businesses had been closed and that there were 70-80 deaths a day – it wasn't uncommon to see people fall over and die suddenly in the street.

Although these reports are terrifying, and similar to stories from other parts of the globe, they're very regionalized. The experience of China as a whole country was, overall, of one which came through a much milder epidemic with a much lower death rate.[3] This is quite strange considering the size of the country and how well populated it was – you would have expected their experience to have been similar to South Africa or India. It has been suggested that Dr Wu's plague of late 1917 might actually have been an early herald wave of flu – perhaps even the original wave (although this doesn't explain the 1916 deaths at Étaples) and that when it returned to China, many people already had a level of immunity to the virus which hadn't been conferred on the rest of the world. This would certainly explain why the southern and north-western parts of China were worse hit – Shansi, home of the 1917 plague, is in the east where movement and foreigners were common. However, without DNA samples from the original tissue Wu claimed in 1917, this train of thought is no more than conjecture. It is also a line of enquiry that would place the blame for the outbreak firmly at the base of the Great Wall, which comes with its own implications in the world of virology. Epidemiologists are still very divided on the question of whether the outbreak started in China and while Mark Humphries in Canada has offered very compelling evidence that shows how the virus could easily have been spread from China in the context of the global military mobilization, Professor Dennis Shanks in Australia makes an equally compelling argument that the CLC men picked the disease up from the trenches and not the other way around.

Whether China was the birthplace of Spanish flu or not, there are other factors that help account for the low mortality and one of them is traditional Chinese medicine and a strong medical tradition in fighting outbreaks. Over many centuries, details about symptoms and how they were combatted in traditional ways were detailed either in writing or through oral histories, passed down through the generations. This meant that in 1918, while still very much closed off to the Western world and its modern, medical ways, China had a great deal of knowledge when it came to outbreaks of both severity and scale – and they weren't shy in applying their learning. Classified as *Wen Bing* (epidemic febrile disease) or *Shanghan* (febrile disease), influenza in its basic form was no stranger to herbalists and healers and they had a tried and tested arsenal for reducing fevers. Focus on sanitation was high and, perhaps most importantly, these remedies were affordable, readily available and widely accepted.

Dr Wu was already working on establishing a modern, science-based and widely available public health system when the pandemic struck. His role at the National Medical Association was primarily about promoting Western medical ideologies and he really viewed traditional medicine as having no value beyond the cultural. Despite his views, he recognized how attached the populace was and so encouraged the dual relationship between traditional medicine and his beloved medical science, so today in China we see a health system that offers herbal remedies and acupuncture alongside the more familiar treatments such as antibiotics. As a Western-trained Chinese doctor, he was in the perfect position to marry these two systems together for the benefit of the country and his role earned him the accolade 'father of modern medicine' in China. In 1930, Wu was appointed director of the first ever National Quarantine Service, designed to protect its borders from invaders like Spanish flu. He also sat on the advisory board of the Eastern Epidemic Bureau. After the Japanese invasion of China in 1937, Dr Wu retreated to the safety of Malaysia where he grew up, but his experiences fighting plague, the 'winter sickness' and Spanish flu have been imprinted on the public medical system in China that he fathered.

Tokutomi Soho sat at his desk in his Tokyo home, pen in hand. It was February 1920, and he had found a quiet moment in the midst of his busy life to write to his long-time friend Yamagata Aritomo.[4] Twice prime minister of Japan and current president of the privy council, 80-year-old Aritomo might seem like an odd associate for 55-year-old journalist and idealist, Soho. But having established Japan's first political magazine, *Kokumin no Tomo* (The People's Friend), in 1887 and the publisher of the newspaper *Kokumin Shinbun*, these strong political ties were important to Soho. Plus, as he had grown older, Soho's views had moved further in line with those of Aritomo. Once a champion of liberal democracy, Soho was now a staunch nationalist – and he felt troubled by the events of recent times.

As soon as Japan had entered the Great War, hardship had befallen its people. While this had brought Soho great sadness, it also made him fearful. He knew from his reading and from observing countries like Russia, that hardship breeds revolution and in Japan the people had been vying for change for a while. That was the subject of his letter today. Arimoto had written to him just weeks before expressing concerns that conditions in Japan might lead to chaos – especially the rising price of rice again. *The rise in prices and the importation of anarchism fan each other ...* Soho scratched delicately into his parchment. *The primary school teachers, the police and petty bureaucrats are budding socialist ... you cannot imagine how much the thinking and ideals of the young today are confused.* So frightened was Soho by his own words, he added, *Please destroy this letter* before sealing it for delivery. He looked furtively out of the window. The streets were peaceful tonight, but who knew what could change tomorrow.

Soho's fears were not unfounded but were based on a series of desperate events in Japan over the previous two years. In April 1918, a strange flu-like illness had appeared in Tokyo and was locally named as 'three-day-fever' – by May it had swept through the armed forces of Japan and was entrenched nationwide. By June it had receded and the people of Japan had bigger worries on their mind. Since the start of the war, conditions had become increasingly worse for civilians and now they were facing a huge increase in the price of rice as demand far outweighed supply. At the end of July, the wives of fishermen in the hamlet of Toyama tried to prevent grain being loaded for export. With the fishermen away for long periods of time, it was the women who had their finger on the pulse of society and the women who also acted as stevedores to load and unload the ships. These protests continued, spreading across Japan and growing in size to include thousands of people – although they were often led by women – through August and September. By the middle of August, a second wave of 'three-day fever' had also begun and this one was characteristically different from the first.

Introduced into a port in the west by the vessel *Hozan-maru* from Siberia, Japan's well-developed railway network made quick work of disseminating the disease to almost every region across the islands. With only 1,237 hospitals and 50,000 doctors for a population of 57 million – that's one doctor to every 1,100 people – Japan was ill-prepared.[5] It's no surprise then that authorities initially faltered, unsure what to do – and they still had the rice riots on their hands.

By the time central government took measures to placate rioters at the start of October, influenza was in full swing. Although there is very little written about the relationship between the riots and the spread of flu, it is not a huge stretch of the imagination to see these large gatherings of people (50,000 had met at one protest in Tsurumai Park in Nagoya in August) as a possible vector for the spread, as we have witnessed in other countries. With their priorities now turned to the spread of flu, the Central Sanitary Bureau of the Ministry of the Home Office tried desperately to resurrect past procedures for similar outbreaks – but an official report notes that no one could remember what measures had been put in place to combat the previous influenza outbreak in 1890 – they were flying blind. Although they sent five inspectors out to six prefectures in late October, they didn't have enough staff to cover all regions and actually had to borrow staff from other government departments to help them assess what was happening – almost three months after the outbreak began. When a severe outbreak was finally officially acknowledged on 23 October, the notice simply urged all those in authority to 'attend to the health of our nation' but failed to offer specifics as to how the epidemic should be dealt with in the prefectures.

Ultimately, the police played a major role in the Japanese relief effort, in spreading information to the public about how to prevent and treat the flu and also collecting statistics on infection and death rates. Most Japanese people would not have seen a doctor and would have been cared for at home, which made statistics difficult to collate and fairly unreliable. As many people in Japan couldn't read the Chinese characters used by the limited number of newspapers available, the prefectures went to great lengths to place posters, illustration heavy with some text printed in 'simple characters' into public places like bath houses and railway stations. In some remote regions, authorities air-dropped leaflets and in the cities, the intermission between films and plays was often used for public talks. However, the focus was very much on self-help and little effort was made to ban public gatherings or temporarily close businesses as had happened in some other countries, although schools were closed in many major cities in November.

The main line of defence was gauze masks, compulsory for the armed forces and police. In some towns, people were not allowed on public transport or into certain businesses unless they donned a mask. It's quite common practice today to see people in Japan wearing masks if they have a cold and it's likely this began in 1918.[6] By early November, the Kitasato Institute in Tokyo was mass-producing an influenza vaccine based on pneumococci, streptococci and Pfeiffer's bacilli which was administered widely across the city by a variety of trained volunteers. While the vaccines would have had no effect on the flu virus, they may have prevented the killer secondary infections responsible for so many deaths in Europe and America. While many people would not have been treated by a registered doctor, traditional *Kanpo* medicine was cheap and readily available and herbal remedies could be mixed at home to keep fever down. Official advice also centred around going to bed and not getting up again until the virus was well past, a recommendation that would have also preserved many lives.

Across Japan, there were major concerns about the price of goods relating to the epidemic, with one company reporting a hike in the price of ice by 60 per cent due to demand for bringing fevers down. In the town of Saha in early November, 500 employees from a local steel works formed a mob and sacked various shops across the city in protest at the high price of cough mixture. While there is limited information available about the impact of Spanish flu on the average person in Japan, stories like this provide an insight into the fear and anger that must have been experienced on the ground.

Spanish flu deaths peaked in Japan in December, with another wave hitting the country in early 1919. Officially, there were over 21 million cases, and just under 260,000 deaths. It should be noted here that some scholars have given the death toll at twice this amount, but they have included a much later outbreak which many believe was in fact a different strain of flu. Despite the slow response from the authorities, and lack of official guidance, Japan's death rate is curiously low in comparison to other countries. In fact, they report the lowest death rate of all the Asian countries during the pandemic. While a definitive theory as to why this is the case has not been developed, it may have its roots in the mild epidemic that spread across the country from April, effectively offering some immunity to the later, more deadly outbreak. The way the deaths were clustered in the more isolated areas that may not have been exposed to an earlier outbreak is certainly telling. This coupled with general good cleanliness, wide-spread mask usage, good quality home-based care and willingness to stay in bed until the fever was gone could explain Japan's relatively light death toll compared to Europe in particular.

In terms of its legacy, the wearing of gauze masks isn't the only influence Spanish flu left on Japan. By 1920, the year Soho was writing his letter, there had been a definite shift in Japanese politics from military to cultural rule and socialist ideas meshed with rapid industrialization. It was the beginning of *Taisho* democracy, a period where the working classes enjoyed a louder voice that garnered more political response than previously in Japan. Electoral reform meant the popular vote now needed to be won and a move toward more socially minded policy, including improvements in health care, began – albeit slowly – at this time. From 1920 until the postwar restructuring of the health administration that occurred after 1945, Japan began adding more services to the public health umbrella, including maternal and child health services and an increase in public health nurses. Ultimately, the strong cultural importance placed on cleanliness, the separation of inside and outside spaces, well ventilated homes and the notion that good health is a collective responsibility stood Japan in good stead during the Spanish flu outbreak and underpins the private and public partnership that sums up health in Japan today.

PART 4

SECRETS IN THE SNOW

WHAT HAVE WE LEARNED IN 100 YEARS?

Chapter 11

Peace In the Time of Influenza

The impact of the pandemic on the peace process
and medicine from 1919

Leaning across the table, sporting a devious grin, Sir Mark Sykes pulled a face and leered, *I'll be wanting one of your eyes! Yes! One of your eyes!*[1] His companion diners, Edmund Sandars, his wife Mary, and Sir Arthur Hirtzel, fell about with laughter at his impersonation of someone they knew, crossed with the story of lunatic inmate who gouged out a fellow prisoner's eye. They all appreciated the joke. *Mark was such a card, with a wicked sense of humour, a rare quality in one who was also so dedicated to his work.* It was February 1919 and Sykes was in Paris, staying at the Hôtel le Lotti in the first arrondissement of the city – but he was not on holiday. An avid traveller who had spent much time in the Middle East, he had been requisitioned as a diplomatic advisor regarding the 'problem' of the Ottoman Empire. Its collapse during the First World War left a political hole in the map, vast areas of land with no clear nation state in place and lots of politicians casting hungry eyes in its direction.

Sykes was both a passionate supporter of the concept of Arab nationalism and a defender of Britain's colonial aspirations and together with overt colonialist Frenchman Charles Francois Georges-Picot, he had tried to marry those two things together in a document that came to be known as the Sykes-Picot agreement. This plan for how responsibility for the Arab nations would be divided between Britain, Russia and France on their journey to self-determination had already come under harsh criticism. The British writer, diplomat and 'Arabophile' T.E. Lawrence ('Lawrence of Arabia') referred to Sykes in his book *The Seven Pillars of Wisdom*, as 'the imaginative advocate of unconvincing world movements... a bundle of prejudices, intuitions, half-sciences ... his help did us good, and did us harm'. Meanwhile, there were those whose suspicion of the region demanded the far heavier solution of full colonial rule. Britain alone had ploughed almost 1 million troops into Mesopotamia, (later to become Iraq) to secure the oil fields, at great cost, and they weren't about to side step the security of that resource lightly. Meanwhile, Sykes' co-author Picot was a supporter of the idea that Syria and Palestine were French and should be under Metropolitan France's direct rule. The draft agreement they came up with was a complex document that had attempted to address the needs and wants of a variety of different interest groups – and arguably failed, especially in the eyes of those who lived on the contested land. Sykes had been a young man, just 36 years old, when he worked on the somewhat idealist draft with Picot that had no Arab input whatsoever. Now, almost four years later, he'd grown up a lot, crystalized his ideas and felt that he could see a path forward – a path that took the Arab desire for independence into account. He was, therefore, in Paris to help with the negotiations, using the document as a blue print to try and achieve a balanced outcome that was palatable to all. But tonight, he was relaxing with friends.

And how is dear Edith? Sandars asked Sykes, as the staff at the restaurant Henri brought over their main course. *I have urged her to keep to her bed,* Sykes replied regarding the health of his wife who had joined in him Paris not long before. *She denied having a temperature, but today had a definite touch of fever.* The conference in Versailles had begun in mid-January, about the same time as the third wave of Spanish flu had taken hold of the city (eventually killing more than 2,000 people in Paris in addition to those already taken in 1918). As it gripped the city in a final encore, it had not spared those attending the conference. Edith had been unwell for several days and Sykes worried about her, but she appeared to be over the worst.

The diners departed, tickets for the opera *Thalis* in hand. A comedy in three parts, Sykes chuckled along merrily and enjoyed a smoking break with Sandars during the intervals. Many other recognisable faces were there and smiling broadly Sykes, indulged in his characteristic showmanship, regaling acquaintances with tales, or engaging solemnly in the talk of what was to come. *And so, I must bid you goodnight!* Mark grinned blithely at his friends as their car pulled up outside of his hotel. He climbed out into the chilly February air and, feeling weary despite an enjoyable evening, climbed the stairs to his suite. In the hall his secretary, Walter Wilson greeted him, but Sykes' usual smile was no longer forthcoming. Suddenly feeling hot, clammy and exceptionally tired, he leaned forward, frowning. *I've got it,* he said to Wilson, darkly, and opening his door he put himself straight to bed.

Over the next few days, Edith nursed her husband herself, convinced his fever was nothing serious. The hotel was obliging, sending up suggested medications and Bovril. But Sykes never got up again from his bed. By the time their family doctor, whom Edith had summoned from Britain, arrived on 16 February, Sykes had a serious case of pneumonia. He died that evening, aged thirty-nine. He was returned to the family home, Sledmere, and interred in the grounds in a coffin lined with lead.

While many mourned the death of Sykes, the peace process, of course, went on without him. The major players in the process were President Woodrow Wilson of America, Georges Clemenceau of France, UK Prime Minister David Lloyd George and Vittorio Emanuele Orlando, Prime Minister of Italy. These four super powers very much controlled the process and met regularly and privately to thrash out among them details of the big decisions before presenting them to conference for ratification.[2] Among those many decisions were the choices they made in carving up the Middle East, creating countries they could control either directly or politically, based on the distribution of resources rather than considerations for ethnic groupings, language, religious affiliations or cultural traditions. The impact these decisions have had since cannot be underestimated, with Sykes' relative and recent biographer Christopher Simon Sykes suggesting that having visited Syria shortly before the peace conference began, Sykes became somewhat disillusioned with the Sykes-Picot agreement and its aims and had shown support for a completely different course of action before being prematurely cut down by flu. Even Sykes' rival and critic, Lawrence, acknowledged in *Seven Pillars* that Sykes had come home from that last trip to the Middle East profoundly changed in his ambitions.

The decisions made regarding the Middle East have come under extensive criticism in the century since and continue to have ramifications in the modern world in which we live. Iraq, for example, is one of the countries 'created' by the peace conference; three separate regions amalgamated into one state under British rule, pulling together not only Sunni and Shi'ite Muslims, but Kurdish hill tribes alongside Christians and Jews. Realising the need for a strong 'local' hand, the British established an Anglophile king, Faisal I, from the Jordanian Hashemite Monarchy, who had helped lead the Great Arab Revolt against the Ottomans. Faisal himself had wanted Syria and had been incensed when this formerly promised land ended up under French control. He and his two brothers had, after all, dedicated themselves to supporting allied forces, uniting their Muslim followers against the Ottomans in order to bring to life their father's vision of a free-Arab confederation. That vision was now being stolen away. But Faisal was out of his depth at the conference, limited by both language and cultural barriers and aware of the mistrust of the French toward him and his people.[3] His delegation was also affected by Spanish flu, with T.E. Lawrence, who was with them to assist, even having to leave the peace negotiations briefly to return to England as his father was dying of influenza. On the ground in Syria and Iraq, the decision to include the French literally caused riots in the streets. After the new map of the Middle East was signed off by the victorious powers at San Remo in 1920, armed uprisings spread across Syria, Palestine and Iraq from July to October with as many as 10,000 casualties. Establishing Faisal at the head of local government in Iraq (and his brother in the buffer state of Transjordan) gave the appearance of offering a compromise in the direction of self-determination, while making sure the seat of power in Iraq would rely on Britain – when Faisal stepped foot in Basra in June 1921, it was his first time in the region and he had no local power base to support his rule.

It's possible Faisal viewed Iraq as a bit of a wooden spoon, but he took up his role with vigour and continued to pursue his passion of a pan-Arabian state. In his pursuit of a better life for 'his' peoples, Faisal achieved many positive things, overhauling the school system and establishing a robust economy. However, before Faisal agreed to the Royal compromise, when he still thought he was going to be King of Syria, he had signed his name in support of the Balfour declaration, also worked on by Sykes – a document Faisal's father Hussein had refused to sign outlining the establishment of a future Jewish state in Palestine. This later formed the basis of the highly-troubled Israel/Palestine territory we know today. When Faisal died after twelve years of rule in Iraq, it heralded a period of turmoil that has never been fully resolved.

The constant echo of decisions made in Versailles about the Middle East, based on a document that Sykes himself had reportedly lost faith in, have reverberated through the whole twentieth century and shaped the short time we have lived in the twenty-first century. The Arab Spring in 2011 was, of course, an attempt to assert self-determination after almost 100 years of complex political interplay with Western powers that had, in some people's eyes at least, not been progressive for the Arab nationalist cause. In turn, those apparently grass roots uprisings brought to the fore ISIL, the Islamic State, whose role in the abject suffering we have witnessed in Syria is beyond criminal. In 2014, when the Islamic State infiltrated Iraq, they filmed themselves destroying the fence at the border with Syria – what they themselves called 'the Sykes-Picot line' in pursuit of their own Sharia law anchored pan-Arab state with no borders.

The peace process was a complex business and the fact that a large number of delegates went down with flu as it played out can certainly be considered a contributing factor to some of the more extreme decisions that made up the Treaty of Versailles. The French Prime Minister was racked with bouts of illness during March and April, while both US president Woodrow Wilson and his closest advisor Edward House came down with flu at the same time in early April. Wilson spent five days in bed before he continued with his duties at the conference and it was noticed that afterwards he was erratic in his temperament and focus, often coming across as forgetful and judgemental – personality traits not in keeping with his usual character. It certainly made him hard to deal with. It has been suggested that he may have been suffering from transient ischaemic attacks, or mini strokes, triggered by the combination of pre-existing hypertension and Spanish flu.

Wilson's bout of Spanish flu also contributed to a stroke the following autumn, the result of which was his premature retirement from public life. This meant he was unable to persuade the US Government to join the newly formed League of Nations or ratify the Treaty of Versailles. The latter is particularly important because, while Wilson, very much the voice of reason during peace talks, had supported wording in the Treaty specifying the fault for the war to be laid at the feet of the German nation, he did not support punitive measures against the German state. With the US no longer part of the process, Wilson was unable to be involved in discussions around the reparations for which the newly formed German Weimar Republic would be responsible and Germany was left having to repay a crippling level of debt set by vengeful European nations who had suffered the most losses during hostilities.

The Weimar Republic was a short-lived democratic experiment that has been described in hindsight as a joyless place whose people struggled despite some positive changes to wages and healthcare made by the new government. A symbol of the German embarrassment over both the fact of, and the outcome of, the Great War, it left little for citizens to aspire to. In order to try and pay the high reparations it had been forced to agree to, the Weimar republic began printing paper money beyond its means, resulting in a currency with no value. Before the war there had been about four marks to the US dollar, but by December 1922, you would need to pay 7,400 marks to buy just one US dollar and the cost of living sky-rocketed. With the value of the currency plummeting, the Allies demanded repayments in hard goods like coal, which resulted in workers in the Ruhr region going on strike. By November 1923, you would have needed over four billion marks to buy one US dollar, and inflation was happening so quickly that money was losing value by the hour. The book *Paper Money* by George J.W. Goodman has some first-person accounts from the time that include a lawyer whose twenty-year insurance policy came due, but the amount was only enough to buy a loaf of bread, and a student who ordered two cups of coffee and found, by the time he had finished drinking them, the price had increased by a third. There are pictures from the period showing people using money for mundane tasks like lighting fires, or children using stacks of notes as building blocks, or to make paper kites. As soon as they were paid, people rushed to the shops to buy things, not because they needed them but because they could barter them for other useful goods later. Possessions had more value than cash.

It was this backdrop of humiliation and desperation, triggered by the unreasonable demands of the treaty of Versailles, that set the stage for the most incredible and damaging rise to power the world has perhaps ever seen – that of Adolf Hitler. He staged his first attempt at power, the coup d'état immortalised as the Beer Hall Putsch in Munich in the middle of the hyperinflation crisis in 1923. Hitler went to prison and the Germans created a new bank with a more stable currency, but the seed of discontent was already sown. Hitler was a very vocal critic of the republic and the nations he felt damaged the people of Germany at a time when the people of the country were vulnerable. It's likely that his support for the otherwise fading concept of eugenics and the idea that the German peoples were genetically superior to those of other nations might not have received such strong initial support in a country that was well-nourished, well-respected and happy. In making Wilson unable to state the case for reason during later debate, the Spanish flu can be seen to be carrying some of the blame for the Second World War.

As Londoner James Shaw, a crane driver at the docks, was walking to work from his Manor Park home in autumn 1918, he realised he felt hot, achy and weary. *It must be this flu*, he told himself as he continued to work. Somehow, he struggled through his shift as the tell-tale fever came on, but he couldn't escape the crushing feeling of inevitability. He had known of so many people who had died from this flu and he didn't know how his daughters, Lucy age 7 and Edith-May just 2½ would cope without him. Even if he were to survive, he would no doubt lose his job while off sick. Some people had been laid up for weeks. With no money coming in, his family were as good as dead anyway. Overcome by a sense of desperate pointlessness to life, Shaw made his way home. Calmly, resolutely, he took his safety razor from the cabinet. He walked to where his daughters were playing quietly. He held them close, so close, so tight … and then took the razor and slit Edith-May's throat. As her sister lay bleeding on the floor, Lucy fought off her father, the man she so dearly loved and somehow escaped, running away with just minor wounds to her neck. Sadly, James Shaw watched her go. Then he took his already bloody razor and with one last glance at Edith-May, ended his own life.[4]

The depression, anxiety and total feeling of helplessness that accompanied the flu in the UK became well documented in the years after the war. Perhaps exacerbated by years of hardship and loss, there nevertheless seemed to be a medical foundation for this exceptional mass despair, which seemed to affect those who had recovered from flu more than the general populace. For soldiers returning from the Front, neurasthenia – shell shock – was a common malady. Today we call it PTSD and symptoms include anger, heightened anxiety and paralysing flashbacks that without proper treatment can prevent the victim from leading a normal life. In 1919, psychotherapy was still a new and growing discipline and there was much confusion about how to treat the soldiers with these symptoms – 'cures' ranged from electric shock therapy to throwing insults about their lack of valour. However, physicians noted that in the numerous patients who had also overcome flu, symptoms also included vivid hallucinations, socially inappropriate behaviour and even a sense of mania about the patient. The poet and decommissioned soldier Robert Graves, who was already suffering with mild neurasthenia when he came down with flu, noted that after his physical recovery from influenza he continued to suffer from severe mental impairment. Strangers morphed into the faces of friends left dead in the trenches, he was terrified of the telephone, exhausted by visitors and would urinate in the street in full public view. At night, his dreams of war were so vivid he would be woken by his own screams.

In their paper in 1919, *Discussion on Influenza*, the British Royal Society of Medicine documented post-influenza patients suffering from depression, neurasthenia and 'nervous' symptoms, which were all neurological in basis. In addition, post-mortems had revealed degenerative changes to the central nervous system in flu patients. Many cases of neurological sequelae – unusual neurological symptoms – were diagnosed after the flu pandemic abated, alongside anecdotal evidence of malaise, low mood and anger among the British population. In the *British Journal of Ophthalmology* in 1920, D.J. Wood described two patients with normal vision before influenza, with a rapid decline in their vision after they recovered from the fever, that eventually corrected itself. In the twenty-first century, we are well versed in the symptoms and occurrence of post viral fatigue and the life-long condition it can morph into, chronic fatigue syndrome, that causes many of the symptoms described by the *British Medical Journal* in 1919.

At the extreme end of the post-viral case load after 1918 are the people who suffered from the bizarre and still not well-understood condition encephalitis lethargica. First described by Austrian neurologist Constantin von Economo and French pathologist Jean-René Cruchet in 1917, this unusual form of encephalitis, also called 'sleeping sickness', swept across the globe in epidemic proportions until 1930 and then, like the flu itself, seemed to disappear. While there have been a few sporadic cases since, it's actually unclear if this very limited number of modern patients were suffering from the same condition. Symptoms included sore throat, fever, double vision, headache, mental confusion and extreme lethargy and could last from a few days to several months. Many patients were left in a catatonic state in which they were described as being conscious, but not fully awake. Some patients would sit, rigid in a chair, unable to respond to external stimulus while others slipped into a full coma. More than half a million Europeans were affected with an estimated toll of five million worldwide. Around a third of patients died of respiratory failure. Out of those who survived, many displayed symptoms of Parkinson's disease[5] (a now controversial observation), while others suffered from crippling depression and extreme apathy that prevented them from living a functional life. Many patients were left emotionally paralysed, living in a 'sleep-like state' for years. Although never fully explained, one suggestion is that it was an autoimmune response to the virus. Others have suggested the two epidemics were coincidental and that modern medicine has failed to determine a strong link. Others have suggested it wasn't a disease at all but the result of brain damage, often delayed, caused by the influenza virus itself in some patients. Von Economo believed that while the two conditions were not related, influenza paved the way for infection with the undefined causal agency of the sleeping sickness.

There were, of course, also environmental factors that caused depression and anxiety in our post-war, post-flu world. For example, there was a global economic downturn between 1920-1, a financial depression which was later dwarfed in memory by the Great Depression of the 1930s. This hit the US particularly hard due to the way the government had handled wartime expenditure. Their Federal debt was significant. Their response was to cut public spending by around 65 per cent, while unemployment was at almost 12 per cent as the country was flooded with troops who no longer had a role in a post-war army. A similar story played out in Europe as troops were slowly repatriated and decommissioned. The combination of economic factors, post-viral fatigue and PTSD cannot be underestimated in the first few years after the Armistice.

As the populations affected by Spanish flu aged, medicine was more able to see the lingering effects of exposure to the disease. A 2010 study by Mazumder et al noted that between 1982 and 1996 in the USA there was a spike in patients over 60 with cardiovascular disease. Further investigation showed that many of these patients had been exposed to Spanish flu *in utero* and researchers concluded this exposure made the cohort up to 20 per cent more likely to suffer with heart problems in their autumn years. Further research into this group also showed that prenatal exposure was linked with short stature and US census data showed those born in 1919, who were prenatally exposed to the vicious second wave, were less likely to do well at school or be able to hold down a job as adults. Studies of other, less virulent, influenza outbreaks have shown prenatal exposure to be linked to low birth weight, diabetes risk and reproductive disorders. Crucially, lab mice exposed prenatally to the flu strain from 1918 showed significant mental impairment and particularly behavioural problems. Other studies have linked *in utero* exposure to flu viruses with schizophrenia and autism. Similar findings have come out of Europe and Australia.

Perhaps the most lasting legacy of Spanish flu is that it barely left a legacy at all. While it has continued to be studied and analysed in niche virology circles, the collective memory seemed to stub it out and hurry to move on. Were it not thanks to a handful of dedicated historians such as Geoff Rice and Richard Collier, who collected personal accounts of the tragedy through the 1970s and 1980s, many first-person testimonies may have been lost. There are a few explanations of this mass memory loss and one of them related to honour. Perhaps in order to dull the painful reality of the loss of a treasured father, husband, brother or son, much pomp was conveyed onto the memory of those who died in battle. Dying from flu, however, did not convey the same sense of honour. In fact, in a world where eugenics had played a strong role so far, it made otherwise brave men appear weak and flawed. A good example of the military attempt to cover up the 'stain' of death from flu is the battle of Meuse-Argonne. Named 'America's deadliest battle' it claimed over 26,000 American sons, while also directly contributing to the end of the war. The battle, and the men who died in it, are celebrated in collective memory. Yet almost twice as many members of the American Expeditionary Forces were killed by Spanish flu, but there are no monuments celebrating their sacrifice. In the French cemeteries where many of those men lie, memorial stones immortalise the battles, with disease conveniently edited out. This of course isn't a purely American phenomenon, it happened across all the armed forces of all the powers. In Germany, it was military practice to give the families of those who died in service a *sterbebilder*, or death card, that would state a cause of death. It was highly unprecedented for any of those cards to state 'influenza', although there are some limited examples. Cards issued to the families of those soldiers who were taken by flu rather than war often stated they died *den Heldentod fürs Vaterland* or an heroic death for the fatherland.

Others have suggested that the influenza pandemic, coupled with the horrors of war and then the extended negotiations and hardships of the new peace, made it all just too much to bear. While memorials, public silences and press interest meant the war became framed as a public tragedy, the personal nature of flu resulted in it being much easier to edit out. Haile Selassie, the Emperor of Ethiopia from 1930 to 1974 and the (very reluctant) Messiah to Rastafarians, almost died after contracting flu in 1918. He never spoke about it and famously dedicated just one line in his entire autobiography to the experience – 'But I, after I had fallen gravely ill, was spared death by God's goodness'.[6] Meanwhile, in New Zealand, author Reina James grew up with her mother, Meg Williams, who she knew was an orphan, but was simply told her grandparents had died from Spanish flu, 'a dull, grey fact'. In an article for the *Guardian*, James herself admits she asked few questions, but as an adult began to piece together the tragedy – her grandmother had died shortly after giving birth to a baby daughter, Christina, a little sister for James's mother. Both girls survived but, weakened by childbirth, their mother succumbed to flu. Meanwhile, serving in the army, their father also died. James notes that while her mother never talked about it, it could well have contributed to her depression and alcoholism in later life. These tragedies, which mostly happened on the home front, were not vague statistics in a newspaper. They were so real, so personal. They were the bodies stacked up in William Sardo's Washington living room, the men who fell to their death in William Hill's lift, the woman who drowned in her own bodily fluids, surrounded by her family in Haskell county. They were the people whose families couldn't afford to bury them, they were the bodies lying at home, waiting to be collected. They were the unborn children of the men at war, the touch of their sweetheart forever taken away from them. Perhaps at the end of it all, it was just too much weight to bear.

Time is a healer, though, and there are lots of good reasons to be interested in Spanish flu now, a hundred years on from the pandemic; to honour the dead, to analyse the medical response, to measure the impact of the virus on the health of the population through the relatively new discipline of epigenetics … but perhaps the most pressing reason for us to remember the outbreaks from a virology, epidemiology, sociology and historical point of view, is because of the high possibility it could happen again.

Epilogue

Northern Exposure

What the bodies in the snow tell us about
the next pandemic

Ebenezer Evans[1] sipped his hot coffee and pulled back the curtain of the school house window. It was 20 October 1918 and Evans could feel the cold coming off the glass. It was about -2°C outside, but thankfully the brazier combined with good boots and thick jumpers were keeping the children warm and quiet while they worked. Looking down toward the docks, his eyes settled on what had made the noise that brought him to the window – the steamship *Victoria* had sounded her horn, signalling that she had arrived in port. With a latitude of 64.5° north, the town of Nome experienced some terrifyingly cold winters, even by Alaskan standards and as the Bering Sea would soon start to freeze over, they would be isolated for many months before the ice and snow began to thaw. The *Victoria* was probably the last steamship of the year and she brought with her supplies, mail and a few visitors from further south to the small 'city' with just over 1,000 inhabitants, give or take.

Down by the docks there was a flurry of activity. 75 people in Seattle had died of flu two weeks ago and Alaskan Territorial Governor Jack Riggs had phoned ahead of the *Victoria's* arrival, demanding port authorities quarantine the ship. An outbreak in such an isolated location would be disastrous. Nome's doctor hurried down to the harbour where he examined the forty odd passengers and crewmen and placed them under quarantine in the local hospital. Five days later, one person had fallen sick, but on further examination it was decided it was tonsillitis, and everyone was free to go. Four days after that, local people started to die. Churches and schools were closed and residents were told not to stray beyond the city limits. But it was already too late. After the quarantine had been lifted, the mushers had loaded up their dog sleds with mail and supplies and headed off on their lonely journey to the north and inland, to where tiny villages of mostly native Inupiat people spent much of their lives entrenched in their own community, cut off from the outside world. When Walter Shields, the superintendent for the region's Eskimo population on behalf of the US Bureau of Education died, Ebenezer Evans was given the job.

The 37-year-old Evans' school room was empty as Nome struggled under the weight of the outbreak, but at least they had medical supplies and a doctor. Evans couldn't help but wonder how the smaller towns were holding up and, as there was no telegraph, he sent a team of mushers on sleds to find out. The report he got back was heartbreakingly detailed. Along the trail to the villages they had passed clusters of bodies frozen in the snow, seen children drifting through the settlements seeking their parents, and found dogs fighting over human limbs. In one settlement, just north of Teller, they found everyone bar a handful of children dead, many dying from exposure as they were too sick to keep the fires going, or prepare food.

In Wales, a settlement about a five-day sled north of Nome, Inupiat teacher Arthur Nagozruk watched in horror as the disease took hold. Death swept the native population and he called survivors into the school house where they huddled for warmth and lived off reindeer broth, waiting for the terror to end. When rescue arrived from Nome three weeks later, they found living children lying between their dead parents for survival and starving dogs eating the bodies that had gone unburied. Three families were completely wiped out, 17 people lost their partner and 40 children were left orphaned. In order to bury the bodies, the rescuers had to lay a charge of dynamite to break through the frozen ground and then piled 172 bodies into a mass grave with some unidentified limbs and body parts they had taken from the dogs. There had only been just over 300 residents of Wales to start with, more than half were now gone. It was the same story across the peninsula. In Brevig Mission, 72 of the 80 residents were killed in just five days. Around 2,000 Alaskans died during the Spanish flu; only 150 were of European descent.[2]

After the virus abated, the people of those northern territories tried to recover. But with many of their leaders and hunters dead, it was hard to find the way. In Wales, US officials offered them a crushing ultimatum – reorganize into new family groups, with widows and widowers coupling, adopting the children of the dead, or see the Inupiat orphans sent south and institutionalized.[3] In 1918, the Eskimos still lived in traditional family units, with generations of oral history and spiritual belief underpinning every decision from who to marry to where to hunt. This began to dissolve after flu; with the native population devastated in both number and belief, their traditional ways started to disappear and other things took their place, less desirable things, like alcohol and violence. Survivors blamed themselves, unable to reconcile that empty feeling inside.

The story of how Alaska, particularly the native population, suffered during the Spanish flu pandemic is a story of desolation, a story of a group of people who for centuries had found meaning and purpose in one of the most challenging living environments on our blue planet and then had it stolen away in a matter of weeks at the hands of a war they knew nothing about and the colonialism they hadn't asked for. But as I am sure the Christian missionaries would have told them in the months and years after the pandemic was over, God has a plan – and indeed it seems Alaska was to play a key part in it.

In the years following the outbreak of Spanish flu, many new scientific discoveries were made which allowed us to understand that influenza was a virus and how it behaved. These were important, because the pandemics kept happening. Asian flu in 1957-8, Hong Kong flu in 1968-9, Russian flu in 1977-8. The discovery of antibiotics in 1928, while having no effect on the flu virus itself, meant that the death toll from secondary infections was dramatically lowered once they began to be used in the 1940s. Meanwhile, good clinical information about the need for fluids, fresh air and bed rest improved the experience of flu for many stricken by both seasonal and pandemic varieties. Researchers across the globe, such as Robert Webster in Australasia and Jeffery Taubenberger in America, made incredible in-roads into discovering where flu viruses come from, how they mutate and the vectors for the spread. In 1948, the World Health Organisation began its global influenza surveillance and response system, (the global influenza surveillance network before 2011), which tracks flu outbreaks globally, identifies possible pandemics and supports affected countries in developing strategy. After the outbreak of Avian flu in Hong Kong in 1997, the rules were changed regarding live bird markets, which Webster says in his book, *Flu Hunter*, he had identified decades before as a hot spot for the inter-species mutation of the virus. However, when the first dedicated Spanish flu summit was held in Cape Town in 1998 to mark the eightieth anniversary of the outbreak, global experts on the topic agreed unanimously on one thing – there was still so much to learn. Not only were the experiences of people across large parts of the globe still missing from available accounts, but virologists still didn't understand why that particular strain was so very dangerous. Other pandemics, while still killers, had behaved more like flu was expected to. They hadn't set off cytokine storms, or undergone sudden antigenic drift, as the Spanish flu appeared to. Without the DNA or RNA from the 1918 virus itself, that question couldn't even begin to be answered.

Since the 1980s, virologists had been trying to get their hands on a sample of the virus. Preserved lung tissue from soldiers who died at the time had proved fruitless, the virus too far broken down from the preservation process to be useful. There had to be another way to find a sample that offered a complete genetic code and in Canada, one group of scientists believed they had it. A team from the University of Windsor, Canada, planned and executed an expedition to the remote Norwegian Island of Spitsbergen in 1998 to exhume the bodies of flu victims. It was hoped that, having been preserved in the permafrost, they would yield a good sample of the original strain. Sadly, it wasn't to be, the men having been buried in too shallow a grave for science to benefit from the permafrost's preservation powers. But after Jeffery Taubenberger published a scientific paper on the partial genetic code, he was contacted by a retired physician in San Francisco with a part time passion for influenza research. In 1997, Johan Hultin had visited Brevig Mission, Alaska, where 90 per cent of the population had been killed by flu, a re-treading of a scientific expedition he had taken in the 1950s. With none of the specialist equipment, team support or precautions the Canadian team had been furnished with for their failed Norwegian mission, Hutlin arrived in Brevig Mission alone, carrying just his wife's pruning shears and a strong sense of purpose. After obtaining permission from the village mayor, Hutlin opened the mass grave he had visited forty years before with the help of four young locals, where they found the victims well-preserved two metres deep in the permafrost. Hutlin extracted some lung samples, placed them in a serum that would kill the live virus but keep its genetic structure intact, and delivered them to Taubenberger by courier post.

On a warm August afternoon in 1978, Janet Parker began to feel quite under the weather. A medical photographer at the University of Birmingham in the UK, she took her leave at the first sign of a headache and put herself to bed. But the headache didn't clear up. In fact, it was joined by a rash and muscular pains and eventually the 40-year-old had to be admitted to hospital, along with her mother. The diagnosis, incredibly, was smallpox,[4] a disease that had gone from affecting over 15 million people a year in 1967, to disappearing ten years later. And yet now, almost a year after the last case had been diagnosed in the Horn of Africa, Janet was symptomatic in the West Midlands – the disease hadn't been seen in Europe for over six years. After Janet died, an enquiry was held to figure out the mystery. Janet's office was near a smallpox laboratory, where tests were being undertaken on the live virus to try to understand it more. While all possible precautions had been taken to keep it in isolation, obviously, something had failed. Professor H. Bedwin, head of the smallpox lab, was so devastated by the error and Janet's death, he committed suicide.

Stories like these are rare, but they still exist, which means the significance of working with a killer virus, and the importance of keeping it contained, was not lost on Taubenberger. In order to fully understand the strain of flu that caused such devastation in 1918-20, Taubenberger couldn't just look at the frozen virus through a microscope – he had to rebuild it like Dr Frankenstein's monster and then bring it back to life. But this was a virus that killed as many as 100 million people, the majority in the space of about six months. The ethical implications of resurrection were huge. The US Government and the National Science Advisory Board for Biosafety (NSABB) eventually gave him permission to go ahead, provided the genetic code was never published (to prevent it being used by others for biological warfare) and that the experiments were undertaken in high-security laboratories by highly-trained scientists. When Taubenberger's team put all eight gene segments of the original virus back together they could immediately see they were handling a toxic super virus – any one of the eight segments when spliced with a more benign strain turned it into a killer. All eight gene segments together were like taking a hand grenade and turning it into a nuclear device. It also proved Webster and Laver's earlier hypothesis that the H1N1 virus originally came from birds and mutated in mammals and helped the science community understand the killer process of cytokine storms. It also revealed that this strain had the ability to block the production of interferons in infected patients, another important part of the body's immune response and another unusual way in which the virus was able to weaken its host. Studying the original H1N1 virus, a piece of research that occurred over nine years, but has proved invaluable to scientists understanding of how these viruses work.

The outbreak of Spanish flu at the start of the twentieth century is considered to be one of the deadliest infections in the history of humanity, affecting a minimum of 30 per cent of the global population, and killing around 5 per cent. In 2009, the outbreak that came to be known globally as Swine flu was also H1N1, showing that this strain still packs a punch and complacency is a luxury humanity cannot afford. Other versions of flu still circulating have the potential to be even more lethal given the right conditions. Avian flu virus H5N1 kills around 60 per cent of people who become infected. So far, outbreaks have been sporadic and easily controlled, but if this strain were to go pandemic we could be looking at a death toll around twelve times higher than a century ago.

Viruses continue to circulate through the human population and between species. They continue their process of re-assortment and antigenic drift and they bide their time, waiting for the right conditions. In 1918, the most virulent flu virus in human history was combined with the most extensive movement of people around the globe and a few complicating factors such as malnutrition were thrown in for good measure and the results were catastrophic. Many believe it is not a case of if but rather when this toxic cocktail of timing, genetics and social vectors will be mixed up again – and on a planet of 7.5 billion people – almost four times as many as in 1918 – with train, car and air travel providing effective potential distribution in short time frames, the impact cannot be underestimated. Our best hope to avoid a more intense replay of Spanish flu is to understand more about what tricks a virus uses to manipulate itself, and our immune system, and learn how to turn them off. By understanding the pandemics of the past, we can safeguard our healthy future.

The killer pathogen that destroys the world is an idea Hollywood is obsessed with, offering us a regular diet of lethal viruses delivered by monkeys that turn humanity into zombies or vampires or time travelling gunslingers desperately seeking answers in the past. In these visions our worlds are empty, barely inhabitable, society and governments have collapsed, and violence driven by survival instinct has become the new world order. But we didn't see this in 1918. We saw desperation, confusion and grief, but we also saw tenderness and a move toward social care. We saw people reaching for each other across barriers of class, culture and language to offer a helping hand. We saw the oppressed supporting their flailing oppressors in the quest for survival and we saw those in power making decisions to benefit the many, not the few in a time when the welfare state was unheard of. One of the key features of the pandemic was the power of collective movements and understanding that, as a united group, this terror was something that could be conquered. While science works to try and prevent such a disaster from repeating, society continues to evolve down the path that was set by Spanish flu, a path where access to healthcare, safe housing and clean water have been recognised as a human right, a path where collaboration is celebrated and a path where group cooperation for mutually beneficial outcomes are seen as the norm. There's still a long way to go before we can celebrate a truly safe and egalitarian global existence, but Spanish flu reminds how much we've achieved already and that achievement is the result of mankind working together.

About the author

J.S. Breitnauer is a British born writer and editor who divides her time between the UK and New Zealand. A graduate in History and Sociology and holder of an MA in Culture, Class and Power in Europe from 1850, both from the University of Warwick, Breitnauer has a particular interest in twentieth century history and the effects of disease and war on society.

Breitnauer has worked as a journalist and editor since 2003, contributing to a wide variety of newspapers, magazines and journals in the UK, New Zealand and the UAE, as well as contributing chapters to two *Lonely Planet* guides and parenting title *Is it Bedtime Yet?* She has also worked for the Anne Frank Trust UK and the Holocaust Centre of New Zealand. In her writing, Breitnauer likes to focus on individual stories that add a personal dynamic to historical fact, to step into the shoes of those who were there and experience a moment of their lives.

This is her first book.

Notes

Prologue

1. Butcher, Tim (2014). *The Trigger: Hunting the assassin who brought the world to war.* p30 Chatto & Windus.
2. McMeekin, Sean, (2011). *The Russian Origins of the First World War.* pp41-75. Harvard University Press.
3. Hastings, Max, (2013). *Catastrophe: Europe goes to war in 1914.* p30. William Collins.
4. Larson, Erik (2015). *Dead Wake: The Last Crossing of the Lusitania.* p28. Crown Publishing Group.
5. Spinney, Laura, (2017). *Pale Rider: The Spanish flu of 1918 and how it changed the world.* p4. Vintage.

Chapter 1

1. Hoehling, A.A., (1961). *The Great Epidemic: When the Spanish Influenza Struck.* p14-15. Little Brown and Co.
2. Grant, Peter, (2018) 'Spanish Influenza in Victoria, Canada, 1918-1920', http://spanishfluvictoriabc.com/spanish-flu-origin-spread-character/how-did-the-patient-zero-story-begin/
3. Spinney, Laura, (2017). *Pale Rider: The Spanish flu of 1918 and how it changed the world.* p176. Vintage.
4. Pettit, D.A, & Bailie, J., (2008) *A Cruel Wind: Pandemic Flu in America 1918-1920.* p63. Timberlane Books.

Chapter 2

1. Taubenberger J. K. (2006). 'The origin and virulence of the 1918 "Spanish" influenza virus.' *Proceedings of the American Philosophical Society,* vol 150(1), pp86-112.
2. Ibid

Chapter 3

1. Killingray, David and Phillips, Howard, editors, (2003). *The Spanish Influenza Pandemic of 1918 to 1919: New Perspectives.* p138. Routledge.
2. Ibid.

3. Chowell G, Bettencourt L.M., Johnson N., Alonso W.J., Viboud C., (2007). 'The 1918-1919 influenza pandemic in England and Wales: spatial patterns in transmissibility and mortality impact'. *Proceedings Biological Sciences*, vol 275(1634), p501-9.
4. Ibid.
5. Killingray, David and Phillips, Howard, editors, (2003). p134.
6. Spinney, Laura, (2017). Pale Rider: The Spanish flu of 1918 and how it changed the world. p3. Vintage.
7. Erkoreka A. (2010) 'The Spanish influenza pandemic in occidental Europe (1918–1920) and victim age'. *Influenza and Other Respiratory Viruses* vol 4(2), p81–89

Chapter 4
1. Chowell, G., et al, (2014). 'Spatial-temporal excess mortality patterns of the 1918-1919 Influenza Pandemic in Spain'. *Bio Med Central Infectious Diseases*, Vol 14, p371.
2. Oesch, D, (2010). *Swiss Trade Unions and Industrial Relations After 1990: A history of decline and renewal. From Switzerland in Europe. Continuity and Change in the Swiss Political Economy*, edited by Christine Trampusch and André Mach (Routledge).

Chapter 6
1. Yang W., Petkova E, Shaman J, (2013) 'The 1918 influenza pandemic in New York City: age-specific timing, mortality, and transmission dynamics'. *Influenza and Other Respiratory Viruses*. Vol 8,(2) p 177-88.
2. Aimone F, (2010). 'The 1918 influenza epidemic in New York City: a review of the public health response'. *Public Health Reports*, vol 125 Suppl 3(Suppl 3), p 71-9

Chapter 7
1. Phillips, Howard, (1984). *Black October: The Impact of the Spanish Influenza Epidemic of 1918 on South Africa*. p15. PhD Thesis, University of Cape Town.
2. Ibid. p14.
3. Ibid. P15.
4. Ibid. p61.
5. Ibid. p152.
6. Ibid. p157.
7. www.theconversation.com/dangerous-echoes-of-the-past-as-church-and-state-move-closer-in-south-africa-65985
8. www.nytimes.com/1985/03/15/world/churches-on-cutting-edge-of-the-apartheid-battle.html
9. Killingray, David and Phillips, Howard, editors, (2003). *The Spanish Influenza Pandemic of 1918 to 1919: New Perspectives*. p212. Routledge.

Chapter 8

1. Tripathi, Suryakant, trans. by Khanna, Satti, (2018). *A life misspent.* p69. Harper Collins.
2. Chandra, S. and Kassens-Noor, E. (2014). 'The evolution of pandemic influenza: evidence from India, 1918–19'. *BMC Infectious Diseases journal,* Is 14, p510.

Chapter 9

1. The first-person account of Ida Reilly and her experiences during October/ November 1918 first appeared in Rice, Geoffrey, (2016). *Black November: The 1918 influenza pandemic in New Zealand.* Canterbury University Press
2. The account of Spanish flu in Temuka, 1918 first appeared in Rice, Geoffrey, (2016). *Black November: The 1918 influenza pandemic in New Zealand.* Canterbury University Press
3. Field, M (2006) *Black Saturday; New Zealand's Tragic Blunders in Samoa.* Reed Publishing
4. http://www.nma.gov.au/defining-moments/resources/influenza-pandemic

Chapter 10

1. Humphries, M.O, (2014). 'Paths of infection: The first world war and the origins of the 1918 influenza pandemic'. *War in History,* vol 21(1). p27.
2. Killingray, David and Phillips, Howard, editors, (2003). *The Spanish Influenza Pandemic of 1918 to 1919: New Perspectives.* p97. Routledge.
3. Humphries, M.O., (2014).
4. Itū Takashi, and Akita, G, (1981). 'The Yamagata-Tokutomi Correspondence. Press and Politics in Meiji-Taisho Japan'. *Monumenta Nipponica,* vol. 36, no. 4, pp. 391–423. JSTOR, JSTOR, www.jstor.org/stable/2384226.
5. Killingray, David and Phillips, Howard, editors, (2003) p68.
6. Killingray, David and Phillips, Howard, editors, (2003). P74.

Chapter 11

1. Sykes, C.S., (2016). *The man who created the Middle-East: A story of Empire, conflict and the Sykes-Picot agreement.* p328. William Collins.
2. Albrecht-Carrie, R, (1958). *Diplomatic History of Europe Since the Congress of Vienna.* p. 363.
3. Sykes, C.S., (2016). pp335-6.
4. Nicholson, J, (2009). *The Great Silence: 1918 – 1920, living in the shadow of the Great War.* p91. John Murray (Kindle edition).
5. Jang H., Boltz D.A., Webster R.G., Smeyne R.J., (2008). 'Viral parkinsonism'. *Biochimica et biophysica acta.* Vol1792(7) p714-21.
6. Asserate A.F., (2015) *King of Kings: The Triumph and Tragedy of Emperor Haile Selassie of Ethiopia.* Haus Publishing.

Epilogue

1. https://www.adn.com/rural-alaska/article/part-3-how-alaska-eskimo-village-wales-was-never-same-after-1918-flu/2012/05/27/
2. https://www.seniorvoicealaska.com/story/2015/04/01/columns/1918-the-big-sickness-spreads-across-alaska/732.html
3. https://www.adn.com/rural-alaska/article/part-3-how-alaska-eskimo-village-wales-was-never-same-after-1918-flu/2012/05/27/
4. Carver, C., (2017). *Immune: How your body defends and protects you.* pp30-31. Bloomsbury.

Bibliography

Websites

www.1914.org/news/influenza-pandemic-in-south-germany-1918/

www.201-1-1%20%20explanatory%20notes%20%E2%80%93%20
World%20War%20I%20

casualties%20%E2%80%93%20EN.pdf

www.adn.com/rural-alaska/article/part-3-how-alaska-eskimo-village-
wales-was-never-same-after-1918-flu/2012/05/27/

www.archives.nyc/blog/2018/3/1/the-flu-epidemic-of-1918

www.bbc.com/news/world-europe-36391241

www.blogs.weta.org/boundarystones/2016/12/21/then-there-were-no-coffins

www.bucknell.edu/about-bucknell/communications/bucknell-magazine/
winter-2017/a-call to-arms/wwi-archives/the-flu-epidemic-of-1918

www.centre-robert-schuman.org/userfiles/files/REPERES%20
%E2%80%93%20module%

www.encyclopedia.1914-1918-online.net/article/alsace-lorraine

www.express.co.uk/news/uk/955767/spanish-flu-first-british-victims-
smyllum-park-infamous-pandemic-scotland

www.fee.org/articles/the-depression-youve-never-heard-of-1920-1921/

www.gi.alaska.edu 'Permafrost Preserves Clues to Deadly 1918 Flu, Alaska
Science Forum'

www.journals.sagepub.com/doi/pdf/10.1177/003591571901200515

www.libcom.org/library/1918-rice-riots-strikes-japan

www.neurologytimes.com/blogs/encephalitis-lethargica-still-unexplained-
sleeping-sickness

www.nma.gov.au/defining-moments/resources/influenza-pandemic

www.openlibrary.org 'The ancestors of Ebenezer Buckingham, who was
born in 1748, and of his descendants', p. 184

www.radionz.co.nz/programmes/black-sheep/story/201856326/epidemic-
the-story-of-robert-logan

www.seniorvoicealaska.com/story/2015/04/01/columns/1918-the-big-sickness-spreads-across-alaska/732.html

www.smithsonianmag.com/history/philadelphia-threw-wwi-parade-gave-thousands-onlookers-flu-180970372/

www.spanishfluvictoriabc.com/spanish-flu-origin-spread-character/how-did-the-patient-zero-story-begin/

www.swissinfo.ch/eng/business/devastation_when-spanish-flu-hit-switzerland/44352910

www.theconversation.com/dangerous-echoes-of-the-past-as-church-and-state-move-closer-in-south-africa-65985

www.theconversation.com/what-was-healthcare-like-before-the-nhs-99055

www.theguardian.com/cities/2018/aug/29/how-spanish-influenza-helped-create-sweden-modern-welfare-state-ostersund

www.theguardian.com/lifeandstyle/2009/sep/19/mother-spanish-flu-orphan

www.washingtonpost.com/wp-dyn/content/article/2006/12/16/AR2006121600408_pf.html

www.wsj.com/articles/book-review-faisal-i-of-iraq-by-ali-a-allawi-1396643621

Periodicals and Articles

Chicago Daily Tribune, 10 May 1903

Detroit Free Press, June 2 1918, p C. 1

The Times, 25 June and 2 July 1918

'Camp Funston', Symphony in the Flint Hills Field Journal. New Prairie Press

AFKHAMI, A, 'Compromised Constitutions: The Iranian Experience with the 1918 Influenza Pandemic'. *Bulletin of the History of Medicine*, Vol. 77(2), p367-392, 2003

AIMONE F, 'The 1918 influenza epidemic in New York City: a review of the public health response'. *Public Health Reports,* vol 125 Supplement 3, p 71-79. 2010

CHANDRA, S. and KASSENS-NOOR, E. (2014). 'The evolution of pandemic influenza: evidence from India, 1918–19'. *BMC Infectious Diseases journal*, Is 14, 2014

CHENG, K.F. and LEUNG P.C., 'What happened in China during the 1918 influenza pandemic?' *International Journal of Infectious Diseases*. Vol 11 (4), 2007

CHOWELL G., BETTENCOURT L.M., JOHNSON N., ALONSO W.J., VIBOUD C., 'The 1918-1919 influenza pandemic in England and Wales: spatial patterns in transmissibility and mortality impact'. *Proceedings Biological Sciences*, vol 275(1634) 2007

CHOWELL G, et al, 'The 1918-1920 influenza pandemic in Peru'. *Vaccine*, vol 29 Suppl 2 (Suppl 2), 2011

CHOWELL, G, et al, 'Death patterns during the 1918 influenza pandemic in Chile'. *Emerging Infectious Diseases,* vol 20 (11), 2014

CHOWELL, G, et al, 'Spatial-temporal excess mortality patterns of the 1918-1919 Influenza Pandemic in Spain'. *Bio Med Central Infectious Diseases*, Vol 14, 2014

DA COSTA GOULART, A, 'Revisiting the Spanish flu: the 1918 influenza pandemic in Rio de Janeiro'. *História, Ciências, Saúde-Manguinhos*, vol 12, no 1. 2005

DASH, Mike, (2011). *The Origin of the Tale that Gavrilo Princip Was Eating a Sandwich When He Assassinated Franz Ferdinand.* Smithsonianmag. com, 2011

ERKOREKA A., 'The Spanish influenza pandemic in occidental Europe (1918–1920) and victim age'. *Influenza and Other Respiratory Viruses* vol 4(2), 2010

HENRY, J., SMEYNE, R.J., JANG, H., MILLER, B., & OKUN, M.S., 'Parkinsonism and neurological manifestations of influenza throughout the 20th and 21st centuries'. *Parkinsonism & related disorders*, Vol16(9), 2010

HOLMBERG M., 'The ghost of pandemics past: revisiting two centuries of influenza in Sweden'. *Medical Humanities* vol43, 2017

HOLTENIUS, J., and GILLMAN, A., 'The Spanish Flu in Uppsala, clinical and epidemiological impact of the influenza pandemic 1918-1919 on a Swedish County'. *Infection Ecology & Epidemiology*, vol. 4 10.3402/iee.va21528, 2014

HUMPHRIES, M.O., 'Paths of infection: The first world war and the origins of the 1918 influenza pandemic'. *War in History*, vol 21(1), 2014

JANG H., BOLTZ D.A., WEBSTER R.G., SMEYNE R.J., 'Viral parkinsonism'. *Biochimica et biophysica acta*. Vol1792(7), 2008

KAM HING LEE et al, 'Dr Wu Lien-teh: modernizing post-1911 China's public health service'. *Singapore Medical Journal*, vol 55(2), 2014

KANG, J., 'A thorough study of the Spanish Influenza: How Japanese party politics and ministerial conflicts reduced the pandemic'. *International Journal of Korean history,* vol 23(1), 2018

LANGFORD, C., 'Did the influenza pandemic originate in China?' *Population and Development Review*, Vol 3, Is 3, 2005

LEE, K.H, WONG, D.T, HO, T.M AND NG, K.H., 'Dr Wu Lien-teh: modernizing post 1911 China's public health service'. *Singapore Medical Journal*, Vol 55, (2), 2014

LUPANI, B., REDDY, S.M., 'The history of avian influenza'. *Comparative immunology, microbiology and infectious diseases* vol 32 (4), 2009

HUMPHRIES, M.O., (2014). 'Paths of infection: The first world war and the origins of the 1918 influenza pandemic'. *War in History*, vol 21(1), 2014

ITŪ Takashi, and AKITA, G., 'The Yamagata-Tokutomi Correspondence. Press and Politics in Meiji-Taisho Japan'. *Monumenta Nipponica*, vol. 36, no. 4, 1981

MCCALL S., VILENSKY J.A., GILMAN S., TAUBENBERGER J.K., 'The relationship between encephalitis lethargica and influenza: a critical analysis'. *Journal of Neurovirololgy*. Vol14(3), 2008

REID A., 'The effects of the 1918-1919 influenza pandemic on infant and child health in Derbyshire'. *Medical History*, vol 49(1), 2005

RICE, Geoffrey, (1988) *New Zealand Journal of History*, vol 22(1)

MAZUMDER, B., ALMOND, D., PARK, K., CRIMMINS, E.M., FINCH C.E., 'Lingering prenatal effects of the 1918 influenza pandemic on cardiovascular disease'. *Journal of Developmental Origins of Health and Disease*. Vol1(1), 2010

Morens, D.M. & Fauci, A.S., 'The 1918 influenza pandemic: insights for the 21st Century'. *The Journal of Infectious Diseases* vol 195,

RICE, G.W., and PALMER, E., 'Pandemic Influenza in Japan, 1918-19: Mortality Patterns and Official Responses'. *Journal of Japanese Studies*, vol. 19, no. 2, 1993

SHANKS, D., (2015). 'No evidence of 1918 influenza pandemic origin in Chinese labourers/soldiers in France'. *Journal of the Chinese Medical Association,* vol 79 (1), 2015

SOLTAU, Colonel A.B., 'Discussion on Influenza'. Proceedings of the Royal Society of Medicine, vol. 12, 1919

SPINNEY, Laura, 'Vital Statistics: How the Spanish Flu of 1918 changed India'. *Caravanmagazine.in*, 2018

STETLER, C., 'The 1918 Spanish Influenza: Three Months of Horror in Philadelphia'. *Pennsylvania History: A Journal of Mid-Atlantic Studies*, vol: 84(4), 2017

SUMMERS, J.A., STANLEY, J., BAKER, M.G., & WILSON, N., 'Risk factors for death from pandemic influenza in 1918-1919: a case-control study'. *Influenza and other respiratory viruses,* Vol8(3), 2014

TAUBENBERGER J.K., 'The origin and virulence of the 1918 "Spanish" influenza virus. *Proceedings of the American Philosophical Society*, vol 150(1), 2006

TAUBENBERGER J.K and MORENS, D.M., '1918 Influenza: The mother of all pandemics'. *Emerging Infectious Diseases Journal*, 2006

WEAVER, Peter. C., and VAN BERGEN, Leo, 'Death from 1918 pandemic influenza during the First World War: a perspective from personal and anecdotal evidence'. *Influenza and Other Respiratory Viruses*, Vol 8(5), 2014

YANG W., PETKOVA E., SHAMAN J., 'The 1918 influenza pandemic in New York City: age-specific timing, mortality, and transmission dynamics'. *Influenza and Other Respiratory Viruses*. Vol 8,(2), 2013

ZHONGLIANG Ma and YANLI Li, 'Dr. Wu Lien Teh, plague fighter and father of the Chinese public health system'. *Protein and Cell,* vol 7(3), 2016

Books

ALBRECHT-CARRIE, R, *Diplomatic History of Europe Since the Congress of Vienna*. Methuen, 1958

BURGESS, Anthony, *Little Wilson and Big God: being the first part of the confessions of Anthony Burgess*. Weidenfeld and Nicholson, 1986

ANTONIUS, G, *The Arab Awakening: The story of the Arab national movement*. Simon Publications, 1939

ARNOLD, Catherine, *Pandemic 1918: The story of the deadliest influenza in history*. Michael O'Mara Books Ltd, 2018

ASSERATE A.F., *King of Kings: The Triumph and Tragedy of Emperor Haile Selassie of Ethiopia*. Haus Publishing, 2015

Board of Governors of the Federal Reserve System, *Banking and Monetary Statistics 1914-1941*. 1943

BUTCHER, Tim, *The Trigger: Hunting the assassin who brought the world to war*. Chatto & Windus, 2014

CARVER, C., *Immune: How your body defends and protects you*. Bloomsbury, 2017

CLARK, Christopher, *The Sleepwalkers: How Europe went to war in 1914*. Allen Lane, 2013

CLARKSON, Leslie, *Death Disease and Famine in pre-industrial England*. Gill and Macmillan, 1975

BIBLIOGRAPHY

COLLIER, R, *The Plague of the Spanish Lady*. MacMillan, 1974

CROSBY, A, *America's Forgotten Pandemic: The influenza of 1918*, Cambridge University Press, 1989

DAVIS, R, *The Spanish Flu: Narrative and Cultural identity in Spain, 1918*, Palgrave Macmillan, 2013

DAVIS, P., *Catching cold: 1918's forgotten tragedy and the scientific hunt for the virus that caused it*. Michael Joseph, 1999

DOBSON, M., *Murderous contagion: A human history of disease*. Quercus Publishing, 2015

GEOFFREY, *Black November: The 1918 influenza pandemic in New Zealand*. Canterbury University Press, 2016

GREBLER, Leo & WINKLER, Wilhelm, *The Cost of the World War to Germany and to Austria-Hungary*. Yale University Press, 1941

HASTINGS, Max, *Catastrophe: Europe goes to war in 1914*. William Collins, 2013

HODGSON, Patrick George, *Flu, Society, and the state: the political, social and economic implications of the 1918-1920 influenza pandemic in Queensland*. PhD thesis James Cook University, 2017

KILLINGRAY, David and PHILLIPS, Howard, (eds) *The Spanish Influenza Pandemic of 1918 to 1919: New Perspectives*. Routledge, 2003

KISHLANSKY, M., GEARY, P. and O'BRIEN, P., *Civilisation in the West, Seventh Edition*. Pearson Longman, 2008

KURY, P., 'Influenza Pandemic (Switzerland), in: 1914-1918'. *International Encyclopaedia of the First World War*, 2015

HOEHLING, A.A., *The Great Epidemic: When the Spanish Influenza Struck*. Little Brown and Co, 1961

MCMEEKIN, Sean, *The Russian Origins of the First World War*. Harvard University Press, 2011

MCQUEEN, Humphrey, *Social Policy in Australia – Some Perspectives 1901-1975*. Ed Jill Roe. Cassell Australia, 1976

MORGAN, T., *FDR: A Biography*. Grafton, 1986

NICHOLSON, Juliet, *The Great Silence: 1918 – 1920, living in the shadow of the Great War*. John Murray, 2010

PETTIT, D.A, & BAILIE, J., *A Cruel Wind: Pandemic Flu in America 1918 – 1920*. Timberlane Books, 2008

PHILLIPS, Howard, *Black October: The Impact of the Spanish Influenza Epidemic of 1918 on South Africa* PhD Thesis, University of Cape Town, 1984

PRICE-SMITH, Andrew (ed), *Contagion and Chaos: Disease, Ecology, and National Security in the Era of Globalization*. MIT Press, 2008

RICE, Geoffrey, *Black November: The 1918 influenza pandemic in New Zealand*. Canterbury University Press, 2016

RICHERT, Dominick trans. SUTHERLAND, D.C., *The Kaiser's Reluctant Conscript*. Pen & Sword, 2013

SPINNEY, Laura, *Pale Rider: The Spanish flu of 1918 and how it changed the world*, Vintage, 2017

SYKES, C.S., *The man who created the Middle-East: A story of Empire, conflict and the Sykes-Picot agreement*. William Collins, 2016

TAYLOR, A.J.P., *English History 1914 – 1945*. Oxford University Press, 1965

TRILLA, A., TRILLA, G. and DAER, C., 'The 1918 "Spanish Flu" in Spain'. *Clinical infectious Diseases*, Vol 47, 2008

TRIPATHI, Suryakant, trans. by KHANNA, Satti, *A Life Misspent*. Harper Collins, 2018

WEBSTER, R.G., *Flu Hunter: Unlocking the secrets of a virus*. Otago University Press, 2018

WEBSTER, Robert G., *Flu Hunter: Unlocking the secrets of a virus*. Otago University Press, 2018

WOODHEAD, L., *Shopping, Seduction and Mr. Selfridge*. Profile Books, 2012

WRIGHT, J., (2017) *Get well soon: History's worst plagues and the heroes who fought them*. Henry Holt and Company, 2017

ZABECKI, D.T., *The German Offensives: a case study in the operational level of war*. Routledge, 2006

Index